### "a handbook of courage, determination, and hope"

*Pressure* is not merely a book about sports. It is a book about life! Sam Rutigliano has confronted the ultimate of life's pressures—and has dealt with them head-on. His story is a handbook of courage, determination, and hope.

>Dick Stockton
>*CBS Sports*

### "a sensitive, emotional narrative"

*Pressure* is Sam Rutigliano's private account of his professional career as coach and his personal life as husband and father. It is complete with on-the-field anecdotes and off-the-field heartaches! This book is a sensitive, emotional narrative.

>Pete Rozelle
>*Commissioner, National Football League*

### "one of the most knowledgeable, caring, human beings I know"

Sam Rutigliano is one of the most knowledgeable, caring, human beings I know. Not only is he a great coach, but a coach that I feel fortunate to have worked with and against. If there were more coaches like Sam, there would be more positive reinforcement.

>Ahmad Rashad
>*NBC Sportscaster*

### "a well-written book and a fine story of a coach's life"

I have read the manuscript of Sam Rutigliano's book *Pressure,* and I found it extremely interesting. Sam is, obviously, a very sensitive, devout, and caring man. I was particularly interested in the early parts of the book that read like a "replay" to me.

It is a sensitive story of a man losing everything that he had worked for all his life. I thought Sam was especially generous in the way he handled it. His caring for others comes out in the latter chapters and in the things that took place during the drug years when he was the coach.

It is a well-written book and a fine story of a coach's life.

>Paul E. Brown
>*Head Coach, Cincinnati Bengals*

### "a warm, personal story about real people"

Sam Rutigliano stylishly captures the exhilarating highs and excruciating lows of life as a football coach. More importantly, *Pressure* tells a warm, personal story about real people, especially how one person's faith in God enables him to overcome the often unbearable pressures we put upon each other. This is an outstanding book about much more than the game of football.

> Tom Landry
> *Head Coach, Dallas Cowboys*

### "the highs and lows, the joy and pain of football"

*Pressure* takes you through the highs and lows, the joy and pain of football. Sam Rutigliano's insights are touched with his own special blend of humor and philosophy. It's a book you will enjoy reading.

> Merlin Olsen
> *NBC Sportscaster*

### "one of the really great coaches of all times"

Sam Rutigliano is one of the really great coaches of all times. His record speaks for itself! I know of no one with any more personal integrity or knowledge to speak about the NFL. His book is going to be one of the most exciting things done in years. His honesty and wisdom are unparalleled. I hope that everybody who has any interest in football at all will read this book. And I know if they do, it will have great impact.

> Bill Glass
> *Bill Glass Evangelistic Association*

### "a remarkable man"

Sam Rutigliano is a remarkable man. Like most remarkable men he brings vast talent and insight into whatever he does. Unlike some I have known, he has the wonderful gift of being willing to share whatever he has or is. He does that here, and I am happy for everyone who will get to know him better.

> Bill Curry
> *Head Football Coach, The University of Alabama*

# SAM RUTIGLIANO

NBC/ESPN TV commentator and former head coach of the Cleveland Browns tells his own dramatic story in

# PRESSURE

OLIVER
NELSON

A Division of Thomas Nelson Publishers

*Nashville*

Published in Nashville, Tennessee, by Oliver-Nelson Books, a division of Thomas Nelson, Inc., Publishers, and distributed in Canada by Lawson Falle, Ltd., Cambridge, Ontario.

Unless otherwise noted, the Bible version used in this publication is THE NEW KING JAMES VERSION. Copyright © 1979, 1980, 1982, Thomas Nelson, Inc., Publishers.

Printed in the United States.

ISBN 0-8407-9087-2

**Library of Congress Cataloging-in-Publication Data**

Rutigliano, Sam, 1932–
    Pressure / Sam Rutigliano.
        p.  cm.
    ISBN 0-8407-9087-2 : $14.95
    1. Rutigliano, Sam, 1932–     . 2. Football—United States—
Coaches—Biography. 3. Cleveland Browns (Football team)—History.
I. Title.
GV939.R87A3  1988
796.332′092′4—dc19
    [B]                                                                88–19537
                                                                        CIP

1 2 3 4 5 6 — 93 92 91 90 89 88

# CONTENTS

# FOREWORD

Sam Rutigliano has collaborated with award-winning writer Bert Akin to give readers a deeply moving glimpse of his life as it has been interwoven with football for the past thirty-two years.

Poignant, friendly, exhilarating, these are some of the thoughts that will come to mind as you read this biography. Football in America is big business and big money—with all the accoutrements. Sam Rutigliano pulls no punches. He talks about drugs, commitment, injuries, losses, and all the other pressures that stem from the football arena. Most of all, he talks about the pressure to win and its effect on men and women, employers, players, coaches, *and their families*.

The author is an open, honest, caring man. As such, alongside the victories and triumphs in his career, he discusses the rough places, the heartbreaking losses, the critical mistakes, and the personal tragedies that have enveloped his family, and how, with God's help, he handles "the pressure."

I'm proud to offer this book to you, the reading public.

VICTOR L. OLIVER
*Publisher*

# CHAPTER ONE

# CRISIS: A SHORTCUT TO MY FUTURE

The pressure started at nine o'clock on Sunday evening, October 21, 1984, with the ominous ring of the telephone in our Waite Hill, Ohio, home. I knew it would be my boss, Art Modell, owner of the Cleveland Browns football team. I had been head coach for that team ever since 1978. Earlier that day we had lost to our arch-rival, the Cincinnati Bengals. When I first joined the Browns, I learned that it was a mortal sin to lose to Cincinnati. Nobody knew that better than I as I walked to the phone, dreading to pick it up. "Hello?" Wrong number. The pressure eased.

We had lost the game 12–9. We blew a chance to pull ahead late in the game when Ozzie Newsome was wide open and Paul McDonald over-threw him. I saw Ozzie break open, and I screamed at Paul. I watched that ball sail right over Ozzie's head, and I wanted to jump up and grab it myself. I almost died. Steve Cox had already made a fantastic 64-yard field goal to tie the game at the half. My stomach pressed up against my lungs. First I wanted to kiss Steve, and then I wanted to murder Paul. My emotions were being yo-yoed all over the place. Both teams were trying their best to give the game away.

Late in the game we had them pinned on their own 15-yard line when Turk Schonert, their backup quarterback, threw a deep pass. It looked like a routine fly ball to a center fielder in baseball. I screamed at Don Rogers, our rookie free safety, whose job was to defend a wide area like center field. When I saw that he was out of position to intercept the ball, I screamed again as loud as I could. I stood there dumbstruck as I watched the ball sail overhead for a completion right at our goal line. The score was tied at 9–9. All they had to do was make a chip-shot field goal to win the game. My stomach was doing somersaults. I was sure

Art Modell's heart was pumping overtime. I couldn't even look up to where he was sitting. I never felt so helpless in my life. How could this have happened? This game was supposed to be the one to turn our season around.

We had them pinned down deep in their own territory, and now suddenly they were on our goal line with only a heartbeat or two left in the game. All of us on the sideline were on our feet, screaming. The players were jumping around and pumping their arms to encourage the guys on the field. Time seemed to stand still as they lined up for the field goal. I yelled again, "Come on, Jim Breech, blow this chip shot, hook the ball, miss it!" I died again right there on the sideline as I watched the ball lift off. As soon as his foot hit the ball, I knew it had hit the sweet spot. It was all over. They beat us 12-9. Now it was Cincinnati Coach Sam Wyche's turn to drink the wine of victory. I was already stomping the grapes of defeat.

On the sideline, I hung my head and thought about all the roller-coaster emotions a coach lives through. Many times, just after a win, you really look forward to going into the locker room. All the joy, the exchanges of high fives, and the postgame press conferences with the reporters from Cleveland and the opponents' cities are sweet indeed. Then we always gathered around and said the Lord's Prayer and thanked Him for keeping everybody safe. We thanked Him for giving everybody an opportunity to express their talents with their utmost ability so they could play from the soles of their feet to the tops of their heads. Professional football is played 90 percent from the neck up. When you're standing in the winning locker room and reporters are asking you all kinds of questions, it's usually fun. You think of things to say much easier than if you've lost that day. But when you lose a game and you start that lonely three-minute walk off the field toward the locker room, a million things go through your mind.

I dragged myself off the field, wanting to get out of everybody's sight. Our record for the season was 1-7. The pressure I felt was almost unbearable. We had lost five games in a row. I wanted to hide, but it was impossible. Like a boxer, I could run, but I couldn't hide. I had to face the music. I had to face the players. I had to face the media. And I had to face Art Modell. The locker room was full of people, but they weren't saying much. The guys had played hard, they had tried, but football is a game of inches, a comedy of errors, and the team that makes the fewest mistakes usually wins. I felt lower than a snake's belly, but I knew I had to say something to encourage the players. I prayed for the right words, and suddenly I thought of Tony Lima, the golfer.

I called the team to attention and said, "Fellas, when I was walking off the field, I thought of Tony Lima. He became a great golf champion, but he wasn't born a champion. He had to work his way through a lot of disappointments. Early in his career as a pro golfer, Tony had the habit of dropping out of a tournament if he felt he had no chance of winning it. He just quit. He would then go to a practice tee and hit balls to prepare for the next tournament. Ben Hogan went to him and told him he couldn't do that. Tony wanted to know why not. Ben said, 'You gotta finish. You can't quit. You can't be a champion unless you finish. You have to learn how to lose and keep going before you can be a winner.' So fellas, regardless of what happens the rest of the season, make sure you finish." It was the last time I spoke to that team. I wondered then if Art Modell was going to give me the opportunity to finish the season.

There I was, in my own family room at home, afraid to answer my own telephone. My stomach muscles almost tied me in knots. The phone rang again. I jumped up this time. I hated the telephone at that moment. I wanted to rip it out of the wall. I knew for whom that bell was tolling. When my wife, Barbara, answered the telephone, I expected the worst. She said, "It's Art Modell."

"This is the Armageddon. He's going to fire me. Firing a coach is as easy as changing a light bulb."

"No, I think he just wants to talk to you about the game. He hasn't had a chance to talk to you yet because he didn't fly back with the team today."

I hoped Barbara was right, but my tense gut told me differently because that was the first time Art had not flown back with the team. As I walked to the phone, I thought about how important this Cincinnati game was to Art Modell.

Everybody knew how Art and Paul Brown felt about each other. After all, Art fired Paul. Paul Brown was the dean of the NFL. Everybody on the Browns staff knew that the two Cincinnati games each year were the most important. I mean *everybody* on the staff knew, from the general manager to the venders in the stands. Art would rather see us rip Cincinnati apart than almost anything else in the world. Like the coaches and the players, he lived and died several times during the Cincinnati games.

We beat Cincinnati in overtime the very first game I coached against them at Cleveland Municipal Stadium in 1978. That's when I realized that the Cincinnati game was something special and that, if I was going to coach the Browns for long, we'd better beat Cincinnati even if we lost every other game.

Back in 1980, just before the Cincinnati game, Art Modell got on the bus and sat down next to me as he always did. It was a must-win game as I saw it. Art put his arm around me and said, "Sam, no matter what happens, we've had a great year." I sat there thinking, *We're 10–5, and we have to win this game to be in the playoffs, win the division, and have the first playoff games in Cleveland since 1972.* There was a lot at stake. If we lost, we would be 10–6. Everybody would have accepted that in July, but we would have been out of the running.

I was sitting there listening to that stuff from Art, who still had his arm around me—I mean we really liked each other. I smiled and said, "Art, you're fulla baloney! You wanta win this game more than you wanta breathe." Art laughed. I said, "It's really gonna be a tough game, but I think we're gonna win it."

That game was a seesaw kind of game with each of us going ahead for a while before the lead would change again. We won the game 27–24 in the final seconds.

In 1984 we were having a poor year. After we lost that game, I got on the bus to the airport with Art and his wife, but he didn't sit next to me. We hardly had eye contact. Suddenly I had leprosy or something. (When you win, the players get the credit; when you lose, the coach gets the blame.) That's when I realized there was no middle ground for a coach. You're either on top of the summit or on the bottom fighting to get back up on top. As a matter of fact, it was the first time that season that Art and Pat didn't fly back on the same plane with the team. Cincinnati was special. You could lose football games as a Browns coach, but you would not be forgiven if you lost to Cincinnati.

There was really bad blood between Art Modell and Paul Brown. No one had been more influential in promoting professional football than Paul Brown, a Hall of Famer, not even Vince Lombardi. Paul started the idea of working coaches all year long. He started the use of notebooks. Paul is the one who started intellectualizing coaching as you see it today. Don Shula, Chuck Noll, Chuck Knox, and Bill Walsh are only a few who came out of the Paul Brown school. So every time we beat Cincinnati, it was another notch in Art's gun belt to justify his firing of the all-time mentor of professional football coaches. I can truthfully say that nothing good ever happened to me during my career with the Browns when we lost to Cincinnati. When we lost that game in 1984, it was the crowning blow for me.

I took the telephone from Barb. I hated the sight of it. I hated even to touch it. Nothing good was going to come from my putting that thing up to my ear. The conversation with Art was short and almost curt. He simply asked me to stop by his house, which was located a short five-minute drive from our home. This was it. I knew it. In the past after a game, win or lose, we always had our postgame discussions over dinner. This time it was the Last Supper, minus the food. As I drove to Art's house, I thought back on my life as a coach.

I had started my coaching career in New York City in 1956. From there I went to Greenwich, Connecticut, then Westchester County, then the University of Connecticut, then the University of Maryland. After that I moved to the National Football League and labored eleven hard years for four different teams as an assistant coach. When I was finally appointed head coach of the Cleveland Browns, my lifelong dream became a reality. In 1979 and 1980 I was voted NFL Coach of the Year. In 1984, my contract was renewed for five years. Now, eight weeks into the season, I was on my way to meet with the owner who was going to fire me. I just knew it.

A few minutes later I drove into Art's thirty-two-acre estate, parked my car in front of the big English Tudor home, and walked to the doorway. Those grounds, that house, always intimidated me a little. Inside me there was still that street kid who grew up in a small apartment in Brooklyn. Sometimes, when I visited Art for meetings, I thought back to our kitchen "conference room" where the family always gathered around the kitchen table. At Art's house we always met in his study. How often Art and I had sat there in those big stuffed chairs, watching football on TV and eating pizza. That study held special memories for me. I could already picture the cozy fireplace area where we had sat many times, savoring a victory or consoling each other after a loss. We had what I considered a special relationship that went beyond that of an owner and a coach. We watched "Monday Night Football" there together.

When we beat Cincinnati in the playoffs in 1980, we settled joyfully in his study. That night 25,000 people had met us at the Cleveland airport. The fans had gone wild. We couldn't go into the terminal. We had to unload at a designated place in special buses. Art and I drank the "wine of victory" together in his study. Blanton Collier, former Cleveland Browns coach, called from Houston to congratulate us as we celebrated. It was the same study in which I met with Art and Peter Hadhazy, the general manager, when I signed my first contract with the Browns in 1978. It was the place where I held my first press conference when I arrived from New Orleans. Now I was headed for that study again, probably for the last time.

Art's son, David, greeted me at the door and led me through the hallway into the study. Art shook my hand and held his eye contact with me to a minimum. He was dressed casually in a pullover sweater, yet he seemed uncomfortable.

We had become close friends. We had encouraged each other as fathers when our respective children had experienced difficulty from time to time. I had sat by his hospital bed for many hours after his heart surgery, the same as I would have done for any close friend, the same as he would have done for me. We had a special relationship, at least from my perspective. How proud I was of him and his position of leadership within the National Football League owners' circle. I liked working for him. I liked being with him. I was very proud of the respect shown him by the public, the other owners, the coaches, and the media. He was, to me, a class act. I was truly proud to be a part of the Cleveland Browns football organization. Art set the example at the top, and it affected everyone in the organization.

Of course, I had been in coaching long enough never to completely forget that only winners ultimately survive. Still, I probably expected more than I had a right to expect. I knew *this* conversation was very difficult for him. No doubt many people would say it's a mistake to get too close to someone you may have to fire or someone who may fire you. I suspected that his message to me was the result of much consultation with the rest of the organization. That really hurt, more than I wanted to admit. It meant that all my friends and associates, or at least all those whose opinion Art had sought, had agreed that "Sam must go."

The dreaded news came when Art said, "We want to make a change. We want you to step aside." That's all I really heard that night. So he believed I was no longer capable of coaching his football team. There were other mumblings about "moving into the front office," but I was too stunned to hear well. The words and emotions had a dreamlike quality to me. I had been a coach all my adult life. It was my career, my life. After twenty-nine years with three different schools, two universities, five professional teams, nineteen moves from house to house, and twenty-three different schools for my children, I wanted most of all to be a successful NFL coach. Now this. The rug was being jerked from under me. We had lost six games. In the final minutes. How close can you get and still not win?

I stood there almost numb, listening to my career as a coach being slammed into a wall. *It's so unfair,* I thought. Even though I had expected Art's words, I almost choked when I actually heard them. I couldn't wait to get out of Art's house.

Just when I was about to leave, Ernie Accorsi and Jim Bailey, both executive vice presidents for the Browns, came in from upstairs. Here we gather at the river. It was like a wake to me, my wake. I felt almost totally isolated. In the past I had been at the very center of the circle of power. All of a sudden, I was being asked to leave. Just like that. Leave. No more discussion. I got the message loud and clear that they no longer had confidence in me. They wouldn't even look at me. I knew how a leper must feel. Already I felt like an intruder. I was just another outsider. I wanted out of there! Finally, I couldn't stand it any longer so I excused myself and left. I wanted to go home.

Back in my car, I drove only a short distance from Art's house and pulled over to the side of the road. A doomsday feeling enveloped me. I didn't want to see anybody or talk to anybody. I just wanted to be alone for a while. A wall of self-pity crashed down around me. Didn't they know what they were doing? The had used me, squeezed me dry, and then tossed me aside. Some friends! What a rotten world. I mean, what did they want, blood?

Wasn't I the same guy who went into the 1984 season being honored by the Cleveland Touchdown Club? Wasn't I the same guy who was praised publicly at that same event by Art Modell who, in addition, chose that event to reveal the extension of my contract for another five years? (How could I have gotten so bad in eight short weeks?) Wasn't I the same guy who had been Coach of the Year two years in succession? Hadn't we enjoyed an average attendance of 79,000 adoring fans at home games in 1979 when we were the Kardiac Kids?

In 1980 we had won eleven of sixteen games, dethroned Pittsburgh, and won our division championship—the first playoff in Cleveland in ten years. I should have known better than to feel secure in the coaching profession at that very moment. I'd had a tip-off, but I had let it go by without too much thought.

That tip-off came right after we beat Pittsburgh in Cleveland in 1980. Everybody went wild as we walked through the stadium. Everybody wanted to slap me on the back and be my friend. But as we walked, Pat Modell said something that pierced through the chaotic joy of the moment. I'm sure she had no idea of the impact her remark would have on my mind. I certainly said nothing about it. But it brought reality to me at least for several moments, even in that moment of sweet victory. Pat turned to me and said, "This was great, beating Pittsburgh at our stadium, but we've just *got* to beat them in Pittsburgh." I should have known then that the life of a coach can never be secure. Maybe NFL owners can never be satisfied with anything less than a Super Bowl Championship. Never quite enough. Always a next quarter, day, or game; nothing that says you finally arrived; always another mountain to climb. In the final analysis, whatever accomplishments you may have achieved, it's always, "What have you done for me *lately?*"

Still sitting in my car that night, I thought that the coaching profession seemed to be an impossible one. You had to be a masochist to be a coach. The news media people would circle me like vultures and pick my bones clean. When an NFL coach gets fired, it's headline news on the sports pages.

What hurt my wounded ego as much as anything was the way in which I was fired. In the past, we had always tried to handle dismissals with great sensitivity. I had personally made it part of my responsibility to guard the dignity of the individual at such times.

I can remember when we were about to cut Reggie Rucker. Rather than do that, I called Reggie on the phone and asked him to come and see me. After he arrived and we talked for some time, he agreed that the best way to handle the situation was for him to have a press conference and announce his retirement. It was done with so much class. That night Barb and I took Reggie and his wife, Carol, to an East Side restaurant for dinner. We talked about what a great career he had enjoyed. We talked about how great it was for him, for Art Modell, and for the Browns to have his retirement handled in such a classy manner. It was much better for Reggie than putting his name on the waiver wire and having some team pick him up for one hundred dollars. This procedure proved to open a lot of doors for Reggie later.

The same thing happened in 1983 to Clarence Scott. We talked to Clarence and his wife, Regina, about his retirement. He wanted to play one more year. I had already tried to trade Clarence but couldn't. Just two weeks prior to training camp in the fall, Art flew Clarence and Regina in for a press conference so that Clarence could announce his retirement. It was done in such a beautiful way. Clarence never played football again, but he left with the kind of class that he showed for twelve years when he played for the Browns. That was the way I hoped they would handle my dismissal.

We had a press conference all right, but it wasn't to send me off with any class. It was really called to announce the appointment of Marty Schottenheimer as head coach. I really shouldn't have been there; most fired coaches never attend such conferences.

I knew it was very difficult for Art. But it was his football team, and his was the only game in town. Professional football is a business, big business. It's easy to say that, but when a coach gets fired—especially when he's had a close relationship with the owner—it's not easy to accept. Even though Art had probably consulted many of his associates, it was his unpleasant task to break the news to me. You can be friends only so long as you win. I guess I forgot that. We had lost to Cincinnati, and that was the last straw. My Armageddon with the Cleveland Browns had finally arrived. I should have remembered that hirings and firings are simply part of professional sports. Maybe getting fired was just a shortcut to my future. But there was much more to the story.

# CHAPTER TWO

# VICTORY HAS A HUNDRED FATHERS, LOSING IS AN ORPHAN

**A**s I continued sitting in the car beside the road, my mind transported me back to the streets of Brooklyn, New York, where I was born and raised. With the suddenness of a modern movie without transitions between scenes, I saw myself as a teenager playing stickball with my buddy, Henry Muller.

I stood in the street at "home plate," which was a sewer cover. I was Joe DiMaggio of the Yankees. How I had loved that man's style and talent. I knew all his moves. Like thousands of other native New Yorkers, I wanted to be just like Joltin' Joe.

I gripped a sawed-off broom handle while Henry fondled a tennis ball he was about to launch at me with all his might. He was Don Newcombe of the Brooklyn Dodgers. He was the enemy. I had watched him many times at Ebbets Field. I knew all his moves, too, and the moves and stats of all the other players as well. I watched "Newcome" now as he glared at me from beneath the floppy bill of his baseball cap. His eyes were narrowed down to slits. I knew his move to first base, the way he leaned forward and stared at each batter, the way he picked up the rosin bag and turned his back on the batter like a matador turning away from a bull. Then he would toss the rosin bag down and whirl around in a crouch to face the batter, ready for the Babe himself. Most important, though, was the way he telegraphed his pitch by spitting tobacco juice. He didn't realize that he usually spit to his left just before he uncorked his fastball. Curves were always preceded by spitballs to the right. This time, the spit squirted left through the gap in his two front teeth. He was going to zing me with his fastball.

Henry didn't chew tobacco, but it was just as real to me as if he did. I wasn't facing Henry Muller; I was facing the big guy himself. Henry *was* Don Newcombe, and I *was* Joe DiMaggio. And I was ready. He glared at me, twitched his head toward first to hold the runner there, wound up, and let it fly. Just where I wanted it. Wham! I caught all of it with everything I had. The ball sailed over the first sewer cover and then over another. Home run! Two sewers always meant a home run. Yankees win again! In my reverie, I looked at my young friend and heard myself say, "Some day I'm gonna get a scholarship to college and play football." And I did.

Funny how your mind plays tricks on you sometimes. As I sat there in the car, I must have switched back from the reality of the present to my early days in Brooklyn three or four times. It happened again.

This time I was back in the locker room at Erasmus Hall High School, one of the oldest schools in the United States. The halls still echo the names of such graduates as Barbra Streisand, Billy Cunningham, Doug Moe, Al Davis, Gabe Kaplan, and Sid Luckman, to name a few. I recalled the day we played before 22,000 people in Ebbets Field. After the game, we were getting dressed in the locker room in preparation for a party. I turned to all the guys and announced, "Some day I'm gonna get a scholarship and play college football." And I did. My mind was really working overtime.

Then, I was suddenly back in a college locker room. I jumped up on a bench and announced to the rest of the team, "Listen, you guys. Some day I'm gonna graduate and go back to New York City to coach and teach."

The guys yelled, "Ha, you won't even graduate!" But I did, and I also became a coach and teacher in New York City.

Still another scene flashed into my mind. I was in Yankee Stadium watching the Cleveland Browns play the New York Giants in the heyday of Jim Brown, the greatest running back who ever lived. I said to my coaching buddies from Brooklyn who were sitting in the stands with me, "Some day I'm gonna be a head coach for a major college or an NFL team." And I was.

Again the scene shifted without transition and began "scrolling" in my mind's eye, as text scrolls on the screen of a computer monitor. Scene after scene flashed past: college football, then pro football beginning with the Denver Broncos, all the years as an assistant coach and then, hey, wait a minute! I *did* become the head coach of the Cleveland Browns! I sat there a few moments after that, and then my mind turned, with gratitude, toward God. I began to pray for help and wisdom. I thought that would be plenty to start with. I was reluctant to pray for patience.

Back to reality now, I pulled away from my parking haven and drove toward home. Something, some mysterious reassurance, seemed to come down around me like a mantle. I felt the Lord was telling me that everything was all right, no matter what the circumstances appeared to be just then. By the time I parked the car in the driveway and walked through our kitchen door, a strange peace had settled in my tormented soul. My spirit was at peace, but my flesh still shook. My ego and pride were smarting. Sure, I was terribly hurt, but I *had* been successful. I remembered that success is always measured in degrees. It's never 100 percent forever. God had allowed me a degree of success few people experience. It's a grand life when everybody showers attention and adoration on you. It's intoxicating. But all periods of intoxication wear off sooner or later, and the hangover comes next. When Peter, James, and John were on the Mount of Transfiguration, they wanted to build three tabernacles and stay there. But Jesus led them back down to the valley where life is lived. That's where I lived, right at that moment. Would I, like other old soldiers, simply fade away? I wasn't ready to fade away, not yet. The Lord had just taken me through a dark time, sitting in the car, and had mysteriously communicated His presence and love for me. I thought, *If God be for me, who can be against me?*

As always, Barb was at the door waiting for me. I looked at my dear wife's face, strained with concern, not for herself, but for me. I was to learn something about my wife in the next few minutes that I simply didn't know before. I said softly, "I'm no longer the head coach of the Cleveland Browns."

"Sam, he couldn't do that! He just told you and the whole world that he wouldn't fire you."

I looked at Barb. There was fire in her eyes as I answered her, "He did, Barb. You gotta win to keep your job."

"Remember when he told that firing a coach in the middle of the season was a cop-out? Did he mean that, or didn't he?" She was really getting hot now.

"You gotta win, Barb."

"Remember when he said he wasn't a John Mecom of New Orleans or Bob Irsay of the Colts? Remember that, Sam?"

"Yeah, I remember, but you still have to win, Barb."

"And then, remember, Pat Modell put her arms around me and said, 'There's nothing for you to worry about.' Remember?"

"Yeah, I remember, Barb, but you still have to——"

"I thought we could believe whatever Art and Patty said."

"So did I, Barb, but——"

"I can't believe they would say all those things to us and then do the opposite of what they said. There's no way in the world they should do such a humiliating thing to you. How can they say everything that's happened in the last eight weeks is your fault? What about the previous six years? Have they forgotten them already?"

"That's football, Barb. Winning cures all ills."

"But Art Modell looked you right in the eyes and told you he wouldn't do those things."

"Look, Barb, I'm not surprised. That's the way football coaching is. It doesn't matter what you did yesterday. It's always today's game and this year's record. You gotta win."

"But, Sam, Art gave you his word. I can't get over it."

"Barb, any owner's word is conditional. You gotta win."

"Well, it's terrible what they've done to you. How could he subject you to such public humiliation? They've been so unfair to you, Sam."

"Barb, you gotta put it behind you. I will, as soon as I can work through it. That's football. You gotta——"

"I know, I know! You gotta——"

"Now you've got it, Barb!"

My wife astounded me. I had never seen her so protective of me. A mother bear could not have been more angry if her cub were in danger. In spite of my own emotional state, I was fascinated by Barb's reaction.

"Sam, I suppose they're going to put Marty Schottenheimer in your place?"

"Yes."

Barb finally calmed down and took a deep breath. She looked at me and said, "Sam, the Lord isn't going to give us anything we can't handle. We've been through worse things than this, and He's brought us through."

I said, "You're right. Even the president of the United States gets fired about every four years. Let's keep our minds on all the good things and not be full of self-pity."

I looked at my faithful, loving wife. How patient she had been with me all those years I had been a coach. I was gone half the time, yet she had always encouraged me. What a gift from God she had been. If I could just soothe my injured ego, I could see this as a new time of freedom. Barb and I would have time together. Maybe God was freeing me to do something for Him. I held Barb close as she gave me a silent hug. A soothing peace settled over me like a cool breeze on a hot day.

The grace of God had helped me survive growing up in the streets of Brooklyn, living many years in the fast lane of professional football, and losing our beloved daughter, Nancy, in a horrible, violent way. I'll tell about that later. I knew then that Barb and I, together with His help, could survive anything, even my Armageddon. But I had a new problem: bitterness. It can consume you like cancer.

One week after I got fired, I listened on the radio to the Browns' home game against New Orleans (television coverage was blacked out in the Cleveland area). My emotions were rattling around in me like crazy. I found myself actually hoping that Cleveland would lose. Can you imagine? But I couldn't help it as the bitterness grew. Rejection works on you like poison. I wanted to erase it from my thoughts, but there was no way.

In the two or three hours prior to the kickoff that day, I found myself visualizing the myriad of details taking place in the locker room. I could see the various players getting taped while some were doing stretching exercises. I watched the clock tick down to the time when I would be giving the last pregame talk and felt my bloodstream surge a little. How can you throw off such ingrained habits in a few days? No way. After living with some of those players for six years, experiencing the ups and the downs, the mud, the bitter cold, the tragedies, the pure joys, the injuries, you make strong attachments that only men in some sort of mortal combat can know—and make no mistake, professional football is pure combat with a little finesse thrown in.

The physical contact is what separates football from other games. A fan sitting in the stands can't hear the impact or the grunts and groans and the popping helmets. But from the sideline you see and feel the physical part of the game. Sometimes you can see helmets with paint scraped off from the contact. It grips you to see and hear it. I kept fantasizing the scene because I just couldn't accept the fact that they were going ahead without me. After immersing my life in that team, building, shoring up, encouraging, sticking with them for six years during which we had tasted glory together, they were throwing me out. They didn't want to hear from me any more. How could Art Modell believe it would be best for the team if I was pushed aside? I felt like a chicken with its head wrung off and its body still twitching. I was still programmed to coach a football game every Sunday. I found myself listening and thinking of things to tell the players, but they wouldn't let me. It was so frustrating. The taste of humiliation clung to the roof of my mouth like garlic.

I thought of Art Modell sitting up there in the loge watching the guy I had brought into the organization, Marty Schottenheimer. I still felt responsible to Marty. I felt guilty about not being there. It was crazy. Rejection is hard to explain, understand, and accept. At first you want to deny that it's happening, but then you begin to realize they've taken the steering wheel out of your hands for good. The bitterness floods in again with each thought. And then the self-pity pours over you like slimy water. For six years during football season, the single most important thing in my life each week had been to win a football game. All week long everything pointed toward it. I built up just the right head of steam, hoping to peak at just the right time. My mind was still attuned to those automatic reactions like involuntary knee jerks. I could no more stop them than I could prevent my knee from jumping when a doctor tapped it with a rubber hammer. Bitterness seemed to be penetrating deeper and deeper into my soul.

I really had no idea how the firing affected the rest of my family at first. Out of the blue I received a letter from Kerry, my youngest daughter, who was away at Miss Hall School in Pittsfield, Massachusetts. It hit me right where I was living. She quoted Machiavelli, reminding me that it's better to be loved than feared and that men are liars and deceivers. *Well,* I thought, *at least she's reading profound stuff.*

It was only through the Lord's help that I was able to work through that rush of bitterness and self-pity tempting me from every side of my mind.

After a week passed, Barb said, "Sam, I wonder why Marty hasn't called. We've been so close."

"He's been busy."

"Marty and Pat have always been special to us. I'll never forget the way Marty drove in from Strongsville to see me at the Cleveland Clinic at three in the morning when I had that emergency. I can't understand why he hasn't called you."

"It would embarrass him to talk to me right now. Hey, if the situation were reversed, it would be tough for me to call a coach I replaced. I can understand that. Besides, what could he say?"

"He could say he knew what you were going through and that he understands. He could say *something* to you."

Marty called seven weeks later. A late call is better than no call, right? But by then, Barb was really bitter about the whole episode.

She said, "I'll never forget what they did to you, Sam."

"Barb, for cryin' out loud, forget it! Let's get on with our lives. Let go of it. You're like an elephant!" And then it hit me. Her feelings weren't for herself at all; they were for me. She's only five feet two inches tall and weighs in at one hundred and five pounds, but I found out she's just as protective of me as Nancy Reagan is of the president of the United States! And, most recently, Betsy North, wife of Lt. Col. Oliver North, stood by her husband, right or wrong, during the intense televised grilling he received from congressmen as the entire world watched. That's love. That made me feel pretty important. I saw Barb in a new way during that time.

The Bible also helped me daily. Barb and I knew it would be our faith in God that would pull us through and nothing else. We weren't exactly whistling in the dark because, by the grace of God, we did have our faith in Him. It wasn't always that way with us, or at least with me. Church was not too important to me during the first twenty-five years of my life. I was a Roman Catholic in limbo, which means that I went to church only when I had to. I'm sure the message was there, but I wasn't tuned in. Even then I didn't see much value in it. But since the church meant so much to Mom, it held some kind of vague importance to me in spite of myself. It was like castor oil to me—I always heard it was supposed to be good for you, but it sure was hard to swallow.

Things of the spirit were a struggle for me during the first seven years of our marriage. Every Sunday Barb, Paul, and Nancy went to Sunday school and church, and I went sporadically to the Catholic church. As time passed, I stopped going altogether. Finally, Nancy asked me, "Daddy, why don't we go to church together?" The frustration was that I had no answer for her. I didn't feel right when I met people and told them my name was Rutigliano, obviously Italian, obviously Roman Catholic, and my wife and children were Lutherans. I just wasn't ready to deal with it.

I run into a lot of people today who have the same problem. Many people approach Barb and me to say they have the same problem of mixed religions in the family. They ask us how we handled it. It has been so rewarding to be able to sit down with them and share how peace came into my life. I have said to many such seekers that God was simply too big to fit into only one corner of Christianity. Although Mom was a staunch Roman Catholic, I always sensed that her great love and compassion for people transcended denominational lines.

While Mom had always urged me to go to church, Dad always urged me to get an education. Dad was an original, a "designer's special."

# CHAPTER THREE

# FOOLS ARE CERTAIN, WISE MEN HESITATE

**M**y father, Joe Rutigliano, came to the United States from Bari, Italy, in 1910. He drove a truck for Ebinger's Bakery in Brooklyn, New York. He amazed me with his strength. I marveled at how he could unload pans of pies piled high. Dad's forearms looked like two Louisville Sluggers. His wrists were so big he needed an alarm clock instead of a watch. I remember one time when Dad was unloading his truck, which was parked on a main thoroughfare. Another truck driver started giving him a hard time. Dad always told me to try to make peace first but, if that didn't work, be sure to get in the first blow and it would be all over. Dad took the driver's yelling for a short while, and then he got mad. I watched his big forearm smash up against the other guy's face. Down he went, out cold. That's how he educated me to survive in the streets of Brooklyn— by example! Dad tolerated no nonsense. He valued education almost equally with religion and probably with as much reverence. He got only as far as the fourth grade, but he had a Ph.D. in common sense.

Dad had an uncanny ability to assess situations and offer advice. He was the Godfather for the entire family. Many brothers, sisters, nieces, and nephews often gathered around our kitchen table asking for Dad's advice. He always had good, sage recommendations for them.

Proud and tough, Dad showed little emotion. He came to America when he was ten years old and helped with the horses his father used to pull his ice wagon. My grandfather delivered ice house-to-house in Brooklyn. Dad's responsibilities included taking care of the horses early in the morning before school. His clothes always smelled of horse manure, and his peers ridiculed him to such an extent that he quit school and never went back. Consequently, Dad always pushed the importance of education to me. Even though he worked very hard, he didn't become successful in his own eyes. It was reasonable for him to assume that his lack of education had caused his problem. He said to me many times, "Sam, you can make a lot of money, and you can lose it. But you can never lose your education."

Once when I was a teenager, he gave me money to put in the collection at church. Instead of going to church, I went with some friends to play dice. What we didn't know was that two plainclothes policemen were playing with us. They had heard about the floating crap game and had been looking for it. It was just my luck to be there when they said, "OK, you guys, you're under arrest." I couldn't believe it when the policeman snapped handcuffs on us. Even worse, in a few minutes I was in a paddy wagon on my way to the police station. This was no stage play like *Guys and Dolls;* this was real. I was in big trouble. I wasn't half as scared of what the police might do to me as I was of Dad. I knew he would kill me if he found out. I imagined with horror his questioning at the kitchen table, demanding the truth from me.

When I finally got home, Dad already knew I was in some kind of trouble. He said to me, "Just tell me da troot, and I won't hurtcha." I thought that was a good deal, and so I told him the truth, thanking my lucky stars for the plea bargain system. The only problem was that Dad didn't keep his part of the bargain. After I told him, he beat the tar out of me. With Dad, it was either his way or Trailways, which meant you were gone. There was no doubt about who was the boss. He was the judge, the prosecuting attorney, *and* the executioner. He told me I would understand better some day when I had a son of my own. My mother taught me all about love and God, but Dad taught me something about the price of disobedience and rebellion.

The apartment we lived in had two bedrooms. One was for my parents, and the other one was for my two brothers and me. We slept together in one bed—which meant we all got the same diseases at the same time. It was very democratic. Sometimes when I walk around on my Waite Hill, Ohio, acreage I recall how we lived as I was growing up in Brooklyn. I think about my own children and how they've grown up in affluence. Sometimes I think maybe they've been cheated. Bill Cosby said it best, "The reason I have disagreements with my kids is because they're rich."

When we were kids, we were surrounded by support groups—aunts, uncles, cousins, friends. It was hard to get out of line. Somebody who cared was always watching. Where we lived there were no baby-sitters. We spent every holiday with the family. I never went to dinner in a restaurant with my family when I was growing up. I can remember how everyone gathered at our home with the women sitting in the parlor and the men playing pinochle in the kitchen. We were always together, doing things as a family, going on picnics, going to parks on Sunday. When I think about all the different cities our kids have lived in and how everybody seems to go their own way, it's no wonder the family structure is in jeopardy. I really appreciate the instinctive love that was shown in our family. We never heard of a psychiatrist or psychologist. We handled our problems without help from outsiders. We did a lot of hugging and kissing and touching. Many times we simply put our arms around each other and said, "I love you." When I think of all the things I've done and all the material things I've acquired, I know there's a void in this kind of life as I look back and compare it with my life as a youngster.

My mother, Mary Rutigliano, worked at Ebinger's Bakery located beneath a second-floor poolroom. I loved to shoot pool with my buddies. We used a code word to indicate we would meet at the poolroom— we called it "the library." Every time I went out to shoot pool, my mother would ask where I was going. I said, "The library." She always believed me and usually said, "That's nice. My son's going to the library to study."

I'm not too proud now of the way I used devious methods to get what I wanted in those days. It was a critical time in my life. The temptation to choose big trouble was as near as across the street from Ebinger's Bakery. All I had to do was walk across the street and go into the OK Diner at McDonald and Church avenues, which was a hangout for local guys like me and gang members who drifted in from nearby.

Three brothers, whom I shall call Eddie, Peter, and Mel, stopped at the diner all the time. When they grew out of their childhood, they were given various names. Pete became Crazy Pete, and Mel became Mad Dog Mel. I'll let you decide what those names meant. Crazy Pete was murdered at a restaurant in Little Italy in Manhattan.

Mel was a classmate of mine at Erasmus Hall. While we were in high school, we used to hang out in the poolroom, play stickball in the streets, go to the movies, whatever. I even dated his sister, Doris. It was strange to me that we took such different paths when we graduated from high school. Mel joined his brothers in the rackets, and I went away to college. Many times in the OK Diner, when I came home on vacation, Mel would put his arm around me and say, "Hey, Rutig, I'm really proudaya. It's great to see a *paesano* from our block make it in da big time." I have often thought that, but for the grace of God, I could have simply walked across the street and stayed. Instead, I went away to college.

I'm sure Mom knew a lot more than she let on, but she treated all my friends as equals. Dad didn't say much, but he knew what was going on in some of the families. He would often say, "I was born at night, but not last night." Dad knew how important it was to mind his own business in those days. If I heard Dad say it once, I heard it a thousand times, "Anytime you have an opportunity to keep yer mouth shut, take advantage of it." Dad was busy taking care of his own family.

Once when Mom was sick, she had to move in temporarily with her sister who took care of her. So my brothers and Dad and I had to get along without her that week. One night when I was leaving to go out with my buddies, Dad told me to be in by twelve. Since Dad slept so soundly, I figured I could stay out later and sneak in without waking him. At 3:00 A.M. I arrived home and tried the front door. Locked. I tried a window. Locked. I tried all the other windows. All but one were locked. Dad's bedroom window was unlocked. Hey, no problem, I'd sneak right past his bed. He slept like a dead guy. He'd never know what time I came in. I worked myself up and into the window. Here's the famous catman, sneaking through the night, eluding everybody.

After about thirty minutes of creeping like an Indian, I got my hands on the floor. Ha, made it! No noise from the bed. Piece of cake. I oughta do this more often. Snap! The lights went on and flooded the scene, hurting my eyes. I blinked, still on all fours on the floor. I looked up and saw Dad sitting by the door with a baseball bat lying across his knees. Along with his big arms, he looked like a bat rack. That was another time he did what his instincts told him to do. He didn't treat me like an illegitimate son; he chastened me, like the Bible says. Actually, he beat the tar out of me again. Dad was an audiovisual teacher. He yelled at me a lot and used a lot of facial expressions when he was "teaching" me. He could stare silently at me and scare the daylights out of me. It's a good thing it was his own son who climbed in that window that night. I'd hate to think of what he would have done to a crook.

Dad taught me many lessons about money. He once told me, "If I have five singles in my pocket, I got no problem as long as I leave um dere. But if some guy comes up ta me and asks me ta change a fin, I have ta take my singles out of my pocket. If I do dat, I might never get um back in my pocket. So, I don't even make no change when people ask." He always believed in "Neither a borrower nor a lender be."

Once my uncle came to our house and borrowed twenty dollars from

Dad. He was apologetic and said he would repay it right away. Dad told him, "Don't worry. As soon as ya can pay me back, just put da money in da cookie jar in da kitchen." Of course, my uncle didn't repay Dad. In fact, he didn't come around our house again for a year. And by that time he had forgotten the loan, but Dad hadn't. He was ready for him. My uncle asked Dad to loan him twenty dollars. Without hesitating, Dad said, "No problem. Help yerself. It's in da cookie jar."

One day Dad came to me and said, "Sam, when you gonna grow up? All you wanta do is play sports. That ain't no way ta make money. Ya gotta make money in dis woild."

"Hey, Dad, I'm gonna be a coach. I gotta prepare myself by playin' a lotta sports."

"Aaah, you can't make no money doin' dat. Ya gotta get a real job some place."

"Dad, if things work out the way I think they will, I'll get all my college money from sports."

"Oh yeah? How ya gonna do dat?"

"You can get scholarships. They pay the tuition, books, meals, everything."

"You mean dey'll pay ya to play wit a ball? What kind of collitch is dat?"

"Honest, Dad, it's the way it works. How else am I gonna get the money to go to college? Lotsa guys from the block have already done it."

"Yeah? Well, I'll believe it when I see it."

"Come on over to Ebbets Field Saturday and watch me play, huh? How about you bringin' Mom? Whattaya say?"

"Hey, you could be woikin' and makin' good money instead of runnin' around in da ballpark chasin' a football."

Not long after that, the recruiter from the University of Tennessee called on us. We sat down at the kitchen table. I watched Dad's face as the guy talked. I was afraid Dad would say something to embarrass me, but he just kept watching and listening. He practiced what he preached about keeping his mouth shut. The recruiter finally finished his offer and looked at Dad and me.

Dad said, "Lemme get dis straight. You guys gonna pay Sam's tuition, you gonna payfa his books, you gonna payfa his food and give um fifteen bucks a munt spendin' money? Fa doin' what, playin' football?"

"That's right, Mr. Rutigliano."

Dad looked at me and said in Italian, "Dis guy's crazy. Some school." Then he looked back at the recruiter and spoke in English, "But what does Sam hafta do?"

"He has to study and work hard on his education while we pay him for playing football."

"Oh, OK, now yer makin' sense. I'm beginnin' to like whatcher sayin' better'n better." We signed for the NCAA scholarship. To Dad, it was a fortune.

That got Dad's attention. He finally saw dollar signs associated with my sports activities. He jumped on the bandwagon. So he started bringing Mom to our football games on Saturdays, even though he still would have preferred to work. It was OK for me to play sports, but he wasn't so sure he should take all that time off from his work. But when we faced off with other teams at Ebbets Field in Brooklyn, Dad and Mom were always there cheering me on. Mom always interceded for me, and I was always allowed to play. Since I played basketball and baseball as well, sports took most of my spare time.

One of the most touching memories I have of my father occurred in 1951 just before I left home to report to the University of Tennessee on a football scholarship. I was excited. Dad was excited, too, but only his eyes revealed the depth of his emotion. I was going to a college that had just beaten the University of Texas in the Cotton Bowl. It was a dream come true for both Dad and me. I had a scholarship in a major college in the USA.

The night before I left for Tennessee, Dad and Mom called me into the kitchen. Their eyes were moist with pride. I knew they had been cooking up something because I had heard them whispering a lot. I knew it had something to do with my leaving for college. For Dad, the pride of that special moment was surely mixed with strong memories of his unfulfilled younger days and those of his father. I had somehow been chosen to fulfill the Rutigliano dream. Joe and Mary Rutigliano's son was to be the first of the clan to go to college. Dad and Mom stood there beaming at me. Then, suddenly it was Christmas and New Year's Eve and my birthday all thrown together.

Dad disappeared into his bedroom and returned with a new suit on a hanger. He handed it to me and spoke in his gruff way, "Here, Son, yer mudda and me wantcha ta have dis new suit fer when ya get to col-litch."

Tears of gratitude welled up in my eyes. I said, "Dad, hey, you shouldn'ta done this. That's an expensive suit. I can get by with sport coats."

"Naw, naw, it's OK. We wantcha ta have it."

"Dad, Mom, I don't know what to say."

Dad said, "Hey, it's no big deal."

Mom hugged me and said, "Sam, you're a good boy. We're proud of you. Don't worry about how much the suit cost. It gives us a lot of pleasure to give it to you."

Dad said, "Hey, Sam, remember ta get da education no matta what else ya do. Dat comes foist, before football, right?"

"Right. Hey thanks, you guys. I mean, wow, that's a nice suit."

It was a gift of monumental importance to me. I couldn't believe it. I was too choked up to say much more. "Mom, Dad, you're the best parents a guy could ever want. I really thank you both." Then Dad handed me another package, a small one.

"Here's somethin' else ya might need, Sam. Open it up."

"Two presents? What can this be?" I unwrapped the package and pulled out a beautiful new wristwatch. It glistened in the kitchen light. It was more than a watch to me. It represented Dad's personal effort and sweat. "Hey, what a beautiful watch!" I put it on my wrist immediately. "Thanks, Mom and Dad. You really shouldn'ta spent all this money on me."

We stood there in the kitchen crying and hugging each other for a few more minutes. I could never say I was not loved by my parents. Italians are emotional people, especially when it comes to their families.

Not until much later did I learn that my father had borrowed the money from Household Finance to buy those gifts for me. I took care of them, believe me. The fabric in that suit was almost like holy cloth to me.

# CHAPTER FOUR

# ENTERING THE FAST LANE

**P**rofessional sports depend on college athletes. College sports depend on high-school athletes. I had to go through the system just as most others did. That journey was not always fun and games.

I had a great year in 1949, my junior year. We won the city championship. But my high-school football career was stopped cold in 1950. Just as I was anticipating my senior year, the New York City coaches went on strike. They were being paid the same as other teachers in the system but nothing extra for their coaching duties. I didn't blame them for striking, but of all the rotten luck for it to happen in my senior year.

Every high-school jock looks forward to his senior year. It's a real high. Things were really buzzing around our school before the strike. We had a dynamite basketball team, too. A lot of our players went on to major colleges. There I was during the summer prior to my senior year, anticipating the glory days to come. Then came the news of the strike. What a disappointment! I was used to playing sports the year around, and now I wouldn't get to play.

That year they didn't award me any prizes for scholarship. I got by, and that's about all. Football was taken away from me, and I got so discouraged that I quit. Who needed a coaches' strike? Not me. I was sick of school, sick of football, sick of systems that wouldn't pay their coaches a fair wage. Nothing was working for me. I just wanted to chuck the whole thing and get out into the work force. When I told my parents I was ticked off enough to quit, they could hardly believe it. But I did it anyway. So what did I do next? Rutigliano the businessman. I got a job delivering telegrams for RCA in New York City. I can remember delivering them on Wall Street and comparing myself with all those button-down-shirt guys. After a few days of that high-powered profession, I began picturing myself delivering telegrams for the rest of my life. I couldn't believe I had taken that job. Talk about dumb. Fortunately, someone else helped me see the light even more clearly.

One day my high-school coach, Joe Monahan, went to Ebinger's Bakery, where Mom was working, to ask about me. He told her how important it was for me to get back in school. Boy, did I play that same tune a lot after I became a coach in high school, college, and the pros! It was because Joe reached out to me that I decided to go back to school. Although I wasn't a model student, he got me all charged up again about going to college, but the coaches' strike was still going.

At about that time, a recruiter from the University of Tennessee came to see me. He had read about our city championship and also about the coaches' strike. He knew I would be very disappointed by the coaches' strike. He came along just when I was most ready to listen and offered something that would be unheard of today. He said the University of Tennessee would pay all the costs of sending me to East Central Junior College in Decatur, Mississippi, where I could finish high school and play football, too. After I graduated, I would enroll at the University of Tennessee. Sounded great to me. How else would I be able to play? I gladly accepted his offer to go to Mississippi and then on to Tennessee. I was on my way. I was back climbing the mountain again.

In Mississippi I experienced culture shock for the first time in my life. In Brooklyn I had grown up with practically every ethnic group in existence. My circle of friends included Italians, blacks, Jews, Hispanics, Chinese, you name it. Now I was suddenly thrust into what seemed to be a foreign country in some ways. I simply had never experienced segregation before. Separate toilets, separate bus sections, separate everything.

It was interesting to watch the blacks come into town every Saturday in wagons. For the first time in my life I saw rest rooms, sinks, water fountains, and seat sections in theatres and buses marked COLORED. There was absolutely no racial intermingling in sports. It was truly like a foreign country to me with customs I had never experienced.

The other Catholics on the team and I had to hitchhike forty miles to Meridian, Mississippi, to attend church. What a difference between Decatur and New York City. You can find a Catholic church about every six or eight blocks in New York, and some of the apartment houses are bigger than Decatur! As an Italian Catholic, I was beginning to feel the same way as the blacks because I had to get up two or three hours earlier than usual on Sunday morning so I could get to Mass on time. At home all I had to do was walk five blocks to St. Edmund's.

In Decatur in those days, blacks always stepped off the sidewalk to make way for any white person approaching them. While we were there, but for the grace of God, we could have started a race riot. Those of us from the North always made it a point to step off the sidewalk first when a black person approached us. We would walk with one foot on the curb and one on the street. Our local friends called us the "short-legged" boys. Just fifteen hundred miles from home and it was like another culture, right in the United States of America! How different it is today.

I went to church out of a vague sense of duty, but it sure wasn't the high point in my week. Jesus was a mysterious "something" who lived in a little box at the altar. We had one Jewish player from Brooklyn named Geroge Birnbaum. When we first arrived in Decatur, a local student asked George if he was a Catholic. George said, "No, I'm Jewish."

The student said, "I know, but are you Catholic?" We probably caused as much culture shock as we experienced ourselves.

You can imagine how the local folks pronounced my name. They thought my name looked like it had all the letters of an eye chart. During football and basketball games, the various announcers trashed my name terribly. The people treated me somewhat as a curiosity because I was from New York City. They called me "Yankee" all the time. Nevertheless, I made many lasting friends in Mississippi. It was an eye-opening education that was to help me later in the National Football League. It taught me how important it was to relate sympathetically to the black players from the Deep South. I talked to many black players, from both the North and the South, who were literally afraid to be seen walking, or even driving, in a white suburb, North or South.

I finally graduated from high school. The name of the school? You won't believe this. Sam Rutigliano, Italian Catholic from Brooklyn, New York, graduated from Newton County Agricultural School in Decatur, Mississippi! I was never even close to a farm in my whole life. But that's football and coaches' strategy. Hey, you take what you can get. I moved on to the University of Tennessee in January of 1951. That was a whole new scene: big-time college football. I never saw so many outstanding football players. They had been recruited from all over the United States. I learned later that good recruiting is the lifeblood of any winning sports program.

I made the team as defensive end, although I had always been a receiver before. It was a disappointment, but at least I would get to play. I had a great spring practice and then attended summer school with two dozen other freshman players. But my disappointments weren't over.

I reported back to the University of Tennessee in the fall of 1951. I was charged up and ready to play. Tennessee had beaten the University of Texas in the Cotton Bowl in 1951, and I was going to be on that same team. There I was with 125 freshmen going out for football. In those days there was no limit to the number of players who could be brought in. I was playing with top players for one of the best coaches in the history of the game: Gen. Robert R. Neyland, Ret., a West Point graduate. He had developed many famous coaches who went on to national fame. All the years that Coach Bear Bryant was at the University of Kentucky, he never beat Tennessee when General Neyland was there. I was living a dream. I hung onto the ball that spring. Hardly any drops. If you want to see a coach get an ulcer, watch his face when somebody drops a pass that hits him right on the numbers. That's a fast way for a receiver to get cut from any team, even if he can run the 40-yard dash in two seconds. You can imagine how happy I was to make that team after all the disappointments I'd had.

But I had another problem. Everybody was getting drafted for the Korean conflict. When spring practice was over, the coaches were fearful about our draft status. Coaches and universities went to great lengths in those days to protect their players from the army draft. They enrolled us in summer school to keep us out of the draft.

When fall rolled around, I was really hyper about getting a uniform on. I was on the varsity of one of the best football teams in America. I couldn't wait. I started playing as a backup behind Doug Atkins, one of the greatest players I had ever seen. Doug became the number-one draft choice of the Cleveland Browns. He was later traded to the Chicago Bears and finally went into the Football Hall of Fame. He was one of the greatest defensive ends of all time. I was all set to play a lot and be on the traveling team, and I couldn't have been happier.

Then the blow fell. General Neyland told me that because I had been in the junior college, it took one year away from my eligibility. If I played during my freshman year at Tennessee, I wouldn't be able to play as a senior. They wanted to "red-shirt" me. All I could do was practice. I wouldn't be able to play in any of the games. Talk about frustration! It was too much. All that year I sat in the stands during the games, knowing that I was good enough to be playing with my friends on the team. It was the pits for me as I sat there watching the team run through an undefeated season and win the national championship. They went on to the Sugar Bowl to play the University of Maryland. I mean, how much can one guy take? But it wasn't over yet. General Neyland retired after that year. I wouldn't get to play for him. After all this being jerked around from one school to another, it didn't work out anyway. I could have died.

When Harvey Robinson, longtime aide to the General, took over the coaching job for Tennessee, I wanted out of there. Harvey was a southerner, and I felt he didn't like players from New York City. In 1952 he told me that I wasn't going to make the traveling squad that year but that there was no question I would be playing the next year if I would just be patient. *Here we go again. Round and round we go,* I thought. That experience helped me relate to football players after I became a coach. I could always understand when a player lamented, "Play me or trade me." That's the way I felt. The coaches kept telling me to be patient, but I couldn't stand waiting. I felt like a yo-yo. *Am I in, am I out, am I offense, am I defense, do I make the traveling team, or don't I? Enough is enough, I quit!* I lived to regret that decision, but I didn't regret it at the time.

Talk about depression! I went home dragging my tail. I didn't want to see anybody or talk to anybody. I knew I had to face Mom and Dad, but I bit the bullet and got it over with. They couldn't understand why I quit college as well as football. There was no way I could explain to them how I felt. How could I tell them that life was nowhere when I wasn't involved with football? Not until I became a parent myself could I understand how they felt.

The last blow came when J. I. Albrecht, the man who recruited me in the first place, contacted me and talked me into letting him call the University of Tennessee. He felt sure they would let me return if I wanted to. It gave me something to hope for once again. I told him to go ahead. Already I was getting my hopes up. Maybe they had come to their senses and realized they let a good player get away. Maybe I would get to play after all.

So, my benefactor called. Then came the bad news again. They said that because I had quit, that was it. No second chance. Talk about feeling rejected. I was at the bottom of the barrel. I couldn't have felt any lower. After all my years of waiting and practicing and preparing myself for football, I wouldn't get the chance. Life was not only unfair, it was stupid. Years later, after I had become the head coach for the Cleveland Browns, I went back to the University of Tennessee. It was not until I talked to Johnny Majors, the present head coach, that I got any peace about having left Tennessee when I was a player. It was a very dumb decision that haunted me for years afterward.

I can remember Eddie Johnson, the starting inside linebacker for the Cleveland Browns who was drafted from the University of Louisville. He was playing behind Dick Ambrose, a guy who didn't have a lot of great talent but was a model linebacker. Dick was a cerebral player from the soles of his feet to the top of his head. Every Sunday he laid it on the line for you, and he danced every dance. I wanted Tom Cousineau, Chip Banks, Clay Matthews, and Eddie Johnson to model themselves after Dick Ambrose.

One day during training camp, Eddie Johnson came into my office and sat down. I saw right away he was depressed. I could tell he was thinking those famous words, *Coach, play me or trade me*. How many times had I thought those same thoughts?

I said, "Eddie, the most important thing for you to do right now is to play as well as you possibly can and learn the game. If you do that, you'll prepare yourself. Then when your chance comes, you'll be ready. Luck is the residue of design. People don't become great players in the National Football League until they learn to pay the price."

Lo and behold, Dick Ambrose went down with an ankle injury when we played the New York Jets in 1983. Dick never recovered. Eddie stepped into that position and now is one of the best inside linebackers in the National Football League. Afterward, as I watched Eddie play, I thought back many times to that little talk we had when he was discouraged. I knew exactly how it felt after I quit attending the University of Tennessee.

One day shortly after I got home from Tennessee, I was trying to make a big decision about whether to go shoot pool or play basketball when the telephone rang. It was Paul Walker, a former classmate at Tennessee, who lived in Aliquippa, Pennsylvania. He wanted me to go to Geneva College in Beaver Falls, Pennsylvania, to play football. Hey, maybe it wasn't all over with after all. I was excited just talking about the possibility. Football was my god at the time. That's all I could think of. I expected to receive all my strokes via football. It was my thing, what I did best, what I enjoyed more than anything else. Without football, life was a drag. There was no thrill equal to running for a touchdown after leaping up to catch a pass and then faking out the defense. I flew immediately to Pittsburgh where Bob Ball, another former classmate, met me at the plane. I was excited. All during the drive to Beaver Falls we chattered about football.

When we arrived, the coach was pleased to see us and invited us to dress and work out with the rest of the team that very day. He arranged for us to attend night classes and work in the steel mills during the day. My friend, Paul, arranged for me to live with him and his mother. I was very grateful and elated. I had a place to live, a job, and an opportunity to play football again. Maybe my disappointment had run its course.

The coach asked us to accompany the team to Grove City that weekend. When we got there, he suggested that we dress for the game just to boost the morale of the other team members. Geneva College hadn't won a game, and there were two "big-time" players from the University of Tennessee sitting on the bench with them that Saturday, ready to go. I always hated the bench. Any player worth his tuition hates the bench. But there we were, watching from the bench, as the game started with Grove City.

The game proceeded to a dull, scoreless tie. Finally the coach came over to me and sent me in on defense. I wanted to play so bad I didn't care what position I played. I was willing to run a towel out to the players just to get on the field. No sooner had I got into position as a defensive end than I saw this beautiful sight, this spinning football, coming right at me. I intercepted the pass, cradled it in my arms like a loving father, and ran toward the goal line. I didn't get to score, but my interception set up the one score of the game. We won 6–0. I was a hero in my newfound home. Things had turned around for me. We really celebrated after that game. I couldn't wait for the next game, which was to be against Washington and Jefferson.

Just as things looked promising, I received another big disappointment. The coaches at Washington and Jefferson had lodged a protest about "the two imported players from the University of Tennessee." Our school administrators investigated the situation, and both of us were expelled because of the way in which the coach had recruited us. Coaches will sometimes do almost anything to win. The pressure is intense at almost all athletic levels—from professional down to Pee Wee football. So, once again I had been cut off from my first love. I was so disappointed that I decided to stay with Paul and continue working in the steel mills. I was beginning to think that my life was jinxed. I worked at the steel mills until Christmas and then decided to go home and wait to be drafted. I was beaten again.

Back home again I heard the same song and dance from Mom and Dad about how important it was for me to get my education. It was like a broken record. But once again I got an important telephone call. Hillery Horne, my former coach at Decatur, Mississippi, called me. It was one of the best phone calls I had ever received. He had become an assistant coach at Tulsa University, and he wanted to recruit me. He offered the usual NCAA scholarship, and so I flew to Tulsa in January 1953. I was back on track at last. I didn't even mind being told that I would have to sit out one season because I was a transfer student. But, can you believe this? The very day I arrived at Tulsa University, my friend and benefactor, Hillery Horne, was fired. Bernie Witucki had been appointed as head coach, and one of his first acts was to fire Hillery. Add *that* to a long line of things I couldn't believe had happened to me!

After I got the news, I went to see Bernie. He looked at me and said, "Who are you?" I spent the next half hour explaining my background and the events that had led to my being there. When I arrived, I thought that I had a place to stay and my meals furnished. But Bernie knew nothing about my scholarship. I got desperate.

"Look, Coach, give me a place to stay for two weeks until spring practice. Then, if I don't convince you I'm good enough to play on your team and get a scholarship, I'll go home."

He agreed, and after three days of spring practice, he signed me to an NCAA scholarship. I had made the team. I felt like I could finally make some meaningful plans. I would finish spring practice, go back to Brooklyn for the summer, work on the docks to keep in shape, and save some money. Things were really looking up. However, if I thought those recent changes in my life were exciting, I was about to discover something many times more important and exciting. I was about to meet Barbara.

How do you know when you're going to meet the girl of your dreams? Do you look out the window and see a star in the East? Could everybody hear the same band playing that I was hearing? I knew she was special the first time I saw her.

# CHAPTER FIVE

# BARB

I was back from Tulsa, living at home during the summer of 1953 and working on the docks as a longshoreman in New York City. One day I was handling large sheets of tin with glistening, razor-sharp edges. Before I knew what had happened, a bundle of tin swung down and caught my left leg, tearing my khaki trousers and ripping a deep cut in my left leg. It happened so fast I couldn't believe it. Blood poured out and ran down my leg. I pushed the wound closed and yelled to my buddies. They rushed me to the emergency room of the Norwegian Hospital in Brooklyn.

I walked in under my own power and saw the most beautiful young girl I had ever seen. She took charge of me, and she was efficiency itself. I realized I was staring at her, but I didn't care. I kept staring. She looked so neat and clean. When she spoke, the sound of her voice got my full and immediate attention. I was so startled and pleased to discover her that I almost forgot about my wound. I noticed the name tag pinned to her white uniform. The name tag gave me the information I wanted to know: BARBARA ABÉ. There was an accent mark over the *e* in her last name. With my brilliant powers of deduction, I decided she must be French. She was a very attractive, petite, wholesome-looking girl with brown hair and brown eyes. There was something special in those eyes. Smitten immediately, I smiled at her and said, "Nurse, I want you to save my leg!"

With friendly efficiency she said, "Would you sit down, please. I have to fill out some papers."

I said, "Hey, I could bleed to death while you're filling out those papers. I might even lose my leg."

She smiled and said, "Please sit down."

It was obvious that she had handled many a guy like me in her capable but very feminine manner. She was nice and seemed out of place in that particular setting. It was a tough neighborhood where all sorts of violence took place during the 4:00 P.M. to 12:00 P.M. shift that she worked. I watched her and felt a strange new feeling of excitement creep into my bones. Who was this girl? Where had she been all my life? Wow, she was beautiful! I couldn't keep my eyes off her. She was exactly the type of girl I had always watched for. Meeting her was the way it must be for a lover of flowers to be walking down a dirty alley and finding a beautiful flower growing out of the asphalt. I had felt "vibes" in response to meeting girls before, but this time it seemed as if the entire band was playing.

Suddenly I realized how I must look to her. I was a dirty, ragged longshoreman. She was used to tough street guys making passes at her. I probably looked just like any other grime-covered guy. Presently the doctor sewed my leg up while Barb assisted him. I was impressed with her professionalism. When the doctor had finished and left the room, she unsnapped a safety pin from her uniform and pinned my torn trousers together. I wanted to keep the banter going, and so I said, "You gave me your very own pin? Does this mean we're going steady?"

She smiled, glanced tolerantly at me, and said, "Whatever." She had heard *all* the lines before.

That voice. That smile. Those beautiful dimples and white teeth. She really got to me. Somehow I had to see this girl again. With fantastic Brooklyn diplomacy and savoir faire I said, "Hey, Barb [in Brooklyn we pronounced her name as *Bob*], whyn'tcha go out with me, huh?"

She smiled again in that efficient but warm, firm, tolerant way and said, "I make it a rule never to date patients."

This time I smiled, "Aw, come on, Barb. I'm not a patient. I'm a nice guy! How aboutchoo'n me goin' out tagedda?"

She kept smiling, but there was a resolve in her eyes that told me I wasn't going to make it with this girl. And yet, I had a strange fantasy that she could one day become my wife.

By the time she had finished bandaging my leg, I knew I had struck out. I wasn't used to striking out. I had always been able to flash my big Italian smile and keep the girls interested. I was picky when it came to females. This one was outstanding, and I was walking away with my bat in my hand and three strikes against me. Defeated, I walked out of that emergency room feeling as if I had been dreaming a beautiful dream that was about to dissolve and fade out forever.

All the way home I thought about Barb. I went into the bathroom and looked at myself in the mirror. No wonder Barb wouldn't give me a date. What a mess! Dirty, bloody, hair messed up. I looked at myself again and thought, *What is this anyway? Here I am getting depressed about a girl I don't even know. What's the matter with me? Hey, she probably isn't even a Catholic. There's no way I could get serious about a girl who isn't Catholic. Mom and Dad would die. The church would excommunicate me. Hey, wait a minute, time-out. I must be going nuts. I don't even know this girl. Get hold of yourself, Rutigliano.*

That night I was quiet at the dinner table. Of course I got a lot of sympathy from Mom about my accident. I didn't tell her about Barb, though. If she wasn't Catholic, forget it.

After dinner I went to my room and stretched out on the bed feeling miserable and getting mad at myself because I felt it was so stupid of me. Maybe I just had a wounded male ego because I had struck out with her. Maybe if she had been interested and responsive I wouldn't have given her a second look. Maybe I was just feeling competitive about the whole thing. I wasn't used to losing. She had beaten me, that was it. *The only thing that upset me,* I told myself, *was that she had beaten me.*

I went out with my buddies that night. In the past, when I had a date with a girl and some of my buddies wanted me to go out with them, it would never bother me to change my plans. I would meet the guys down on the corner and we'd talk about everything guys talk about, which is girls mostly.

On this particular night, I was hanging around the corner with the guys and all I could think about was Barb. She was filling my thoughts, and somehow I didn't like it. I didn't like the feeling of losing control of myself. All the time I'm with the guys I'm thinking, *Hey, what am I doing with these guys when I could be with a fantastic girl like Barb?* Some of us are slow learners! I knew then that I'd rather be with her than anybody.

Before I met Barb I thought of girls as being as plentiful as buses. If I missed one, another one would come along soon. I didn't feel that way about Barb. No other girl had ever gotten to me like this before.

I finally decided to go home and go to bed. My wound was hurting a little anyway, and I wanted to go to sleep and forget the entire day. It had been a bust all the way around.

When I arrived at home later, Mom met me and said, "Sam, some cute-sounding nurse called from the hospital and left this number for you to call."

My adrenaline spurted as I took the note from Mom. I felt like I just made a shot at the final buzzer and won the game. *All right!* She was impressed after all. She was probably calling to say she was sorry for turning me down. She probably wanted me to take her out so we could get acquainted.

Mom smiled at me and said, "She wants you to call her at the hospital in the morning."

Acting almost bored, I cooled it in front of Mom. I tried to hide my excitement as I said, "Thanks. Yeah, I'll call her in the morning. G'night, Mom." I turned to go to my room and then the blow came.

Mom's next words gave me the same feeling I had once when I thought I had run for a touchdown only to hear the referee call the play back because I had stepped out of bounds on the sideline. "She said she needs some more information about your insurance."

*Fumble,* I thought. Dejected, I said, "Yeah. Thanks, Mom." I went to my room and emptied my pockets on the dresser. When I took my trousers off, I stood there holding them and stared at that safety pin Barb had given me. I can't tell you why I gently unpinned it and slipped it into my wallet. What was I trying to hold onto? Why was I doing something so dumb and sentimental?

The next day I had worked up a degree of new hope before I called her. Sure enough, all she wanted was the insurance information. I mean, that's *all* she wanted, nothing more. But here was my chance, maybe my last chance, so I bored in.

"Hey look, Barb, gimme a break. I'm a nice guy, really I am. I just want to get to know you." I tried flattery, "I think you're a terrific girl." I tried humor, "So you're not Italian. I can make allowances!"

"Mr. Rutigliano, I'm sorry, but I just never date patients. It's always been my policy."

"Hey, I can understand that. It's always been my policy never to date nurses, but this time I'm willing to make an exception."

At least she hadn't hung up yet. But she wouldn't budge. "Mr. Rutigliano, I do appreciate your interest, but I just don't think I should break the rules."

"Whose rules, Barb? Your rules or the hospital's? And since we have a relationship now, please call me Sam."

"Really, Sam, it just isn't a good idea."

"I wanta tell you something, Barb, you're the most terrific girl I ever saw. You probably think I always look the way I did when you saw me in my work clothes. Hey, listen, I clean up nice! You oughta see me in a nice suit. Besides, my intentions are honorable. How about if I just come over to see you all dressed up so you can see what a nice guy I am?"

She still wouldn't budge, and we finally said good-bye. But I couldn't get that girl off my mind. I was determined to keep after her until she went out with me. All that day I kept calling her. At least she didn't get mad and hang up on me. I wore her down. She reluctantly agreed to a date. The next Sunday I would pick her up at her residence in the Bay Ridge section of Brooklyn. She gave me her address, and I was singing inside for the rest of the day because the full band was playing.

I hung up the phone and thought of the safety pin in my wallet. Why had I done that? The guys would kid me unmercifully if they knew about it. How could I have known then that Barb's little safety pin, painted with red fingernail polish for identification, would remain in my wallet for the next thirty-two years to this very day?

# CHAPTER SIX

# WE TOSS THE COIN, GOD MAKES THE DECISION

**B**arb had told me she lived with three other young women. When I arrived at the address she had given me, I thought there must be a mistake. A young woman answered the door and invited me in. Inside I saw a dozen young men and women sitting in what appeared to be a doctor's waiting room. They were all quietly reading books. *So,* I thought, *Barb's father is a doctor, and all these people are his patients. Maybe he specializes in young people or something.* No one paid much attention to me as I quietly found a seat. It was confusing to me because I didn't see a receptionist or a nurse or even a desk. I thumbed through a magazine and waited. I kept looking at my watch as the minutes ticked by. No response from Barb or anyone else for that matter. I soon realized that the young people were part of a church group having some kind of social evening together. Right away I was uncomfortable because I usually kept my distance from those types. I just kept my nose stuck in the magazine, wondering where Barb was.

After forty-five minutes, Barb came out. It was worth the wait. She looked gorgeous. Her eyes lit up like diamonds when she spoke, "Oh, Sam, I'm very sorry I'm so late. I completely forgot you were coming."

I didn't want to let my wounded ego show, and I played it cool. "So, how ya been?"

"Fine. Working hard at the hospital. How's your leg?"

"Great. You did a good job. You saved my leg, Barb."

"I'm glad it's all right. That was a nasty cut. By the way, ah, Sam, where are we going tonight?" She didn't make any move toward the door.

"Oh, wherever you want."

"But don't you have something in mind, a movie or something?"

I suddenly realized she was uneasy about going out with me. I tried to put her at ease. "Hey, Barb, we'll go wherever you want. You wanta see a movie?"

"That would be nice. Which one did you have in mind?"

"There's a terrific movie playing with Clark Gable and Gene Tierney."

"Oh good, you must mean *Never Let Me Go*."

"Yeah, that's it." Being with her and talking with her had already caused me to forget how late she had been. For the first time in my life I was totally content just being with a girl—this girl. There was absolutely nothing else I wanted to do.

She turned back to the door she had come out of and said, "Excuse me a minute." She was gone for just a couple of minutes and then reappeared. "I'm ready now, Sam. Let's go."

We walked to the subway to go to the Metropolitan Theatre in downtown Brooklyn. I had a strong awareness that there was something special about Barb. I wasn't quite sure what it was yet, but I was sure it wasn't my imagination. It was affecting me very strongly. I mean, this wasn't just any pushover of a girl who was boy crazy. Although I couldn't pin it down, I found myself poised to respect her. I knew this date was some kind of mysterious meeting. I felt responsible for taking care of her while she was with me out on the streets. I hadn't felt that protective toward a girl before. I sensed this in myself while at the same time I knew it wasn't just a brotherly feeling. This was Romeo and Juliet, Mickey Rooney and Judy Garland. Man, this was romance. I hadn't even held Barb's hand yet. What had gotten into me?

Inside the theatre we found seats in the dark. We didn't talk much during the movie. But I had feelings ricocheting all over the walls of that movie house. Old Clark was smooth and confident of himself. Man, he was the varsity. I felt like a second-stringer. The movie was a love story that both Barb and I were caught up in.

About halfway through the movie, I was *really* getting into it. Old Clark was leading the way. Suddenly he was my model. Just as I used to fantasize about being Joe DiMaggio, I was now Clark Gable himself. His vibes had infiltrated into mine. My confidence was high. With no further hesitation, I made my move and took her hand in mine. My beachhead was established. When I think of how ludicrous that must sound today, I have to laugh. But then, it was real, I mean real. Her hand and mine. Something *real* was happening. Never mind the movie. It was only a movie. But this special girl had my heart pumping. *Hey*, I thought to myself, *hadn't I dated plenty of girls before her and never felt this way? How many times had I taken a girl to the back seats of a movie theatre just to smooch?* This time I found myself acting like a young guy on his very first date ever. I found myself really caring how this girl would respond to me. I wanted her to like me almost more than anything else right then. I gently squeezed her hand. Time seemed to stop. I almost held my breath like a man who hadn't been close to a female for years. She squeezed back. Contact was made! I felt the sparks. She felt the sparks. This might be it, the real thing, and I didn't mean Coca-Cola.

When I was out with other girls, I usually thought nothing of putting my arm around my date and smooching during the movie. Barb was the first girl I dated who caused me to go slow with the physical stuff. I had an inner feeling of really being respectful but comfortable around her, even though it was our first date.

When the movie ended, it was obvious to both of us that we really enjoyed each other's company. As we began to share our thoughts, we discovered a common love for Chinese food so we found a Chinese restaurant in downtown Brooklyn. After we ordered, Barb excused herself and left the table. I didn't think much about it until half an hour later when she left the table again. When I asked her about it, I began to learn how honest Barb could be.

"You know, Sam, I have a confession to make to you. I really didn't want to go out with you. I didn't know anything about you, where you came from, or what your real motives were. The only reason I decided to take a chance on you was because you said your intentions were honorable. I never had a guy say that to me before. As for my leaving the table so much, I've been reporting my whereabouts to my girlfriend about every half hour."

"Yeah?"

"In fact, up until two hours before you came to our apartment, I had forgotten all about our date. I think I agreed to go out with you just to get you to hang up the phone."

"Hey, Barb, I can understand how you must have felt. I looked terrible when we first met. Now I have a confession to make to you. I'm not a longshoreman. I'm in my third year at Tulsa University. My uncle is a foreman on the docks, and he was kind enough to give me a job during the summer. He's a great guy, and I've learned a lot from him. I'm only working there for the summer. Besides, it keeps me in shape. I'm into sports pretty heavy."

"Oh, so you're a college student. What are you majoring in?"

"Education. I'm planning to be a coach and a teacher."

"That's nice. In Germany teachers are highly respected."

"I wish it was that way in this country. Are you from Germany?"

"I was born in this country, but I lived in Germany for several years. My parents are natives of Germany."

I could see relief coming into her face almost as if the news about my education was something she had hoped for. Although the evening was still early, I wanted to book another date with her right away. We talked during the entire dinner and then walked and talked for hours. Time passed so quickly. I had never been around any girl who attracted me more than Barb. Before meeting her, I always preferred to go out with my buddies rather than have a date. Of course, I was usually broke, and that had a lot to do with it, too. I never got too serious with any girl before that. But I don't believe that anything or anyone could have pulled me away from Barb. It seemed as if we walked all over Brooklyn that evening, and she poured her life story to me. Man, was I interested.

"Sam, you couldn't image how thoroughly Dresden was destroyed during the war. The funny thing was that I was an American citizen all during that time from 1937 to 1946. Everything was bombed out. We had no food, water was scarce, we scavenged through fields and barns. If we found an egg somewhere, it was like a steak to us. But, because my sister and I were American citizens, my dad could ride a train from Dresden to Berlin to pick up food from the United Nations Relief Association for us. Meantime the Communists were taking over East Germany, and Dad was worried about us. If we didn't go back to the States before our sixteenth birthdays, we would lose our American citizenship. So Dad finally decided we should leave Germany and return to America. But my parents stayed in Germany."

"That must have been a hard thing for all of you, huh?"

"Yes. But we did it, and fortunately that's when we met Pastor and Mrs. Paul Pallmeyer through the Lutheran Aid Society. They practically adopted me, and they treated me as their own daughter."

Fascinated, I listened to this beautiful, bright girl as she told me her story. Her face was so animated, and her eyes sparkled as she talked. She was full of life, and I knew something was happening to me I might never be able to stop. I knew I didn't want to stop whatever it was that was happening. I loved it. It was even better than football! I stared at her until she had finished her story. I'm a talker, yet I was quite content to listen to Barb.

We returned to her apartment that night and talked and smooched on the front porch. It seemed as if we had known each other for a decade. I didn't want the evening to end. Eventually, we both had to get ready for work. I had to grab a cab, which I couldn't afford, get home, change clothes, and go to work on the docks. Neither of us got any sleep that night.

Something special had started clicking between us on our date that night. We dated steadily during the summer of 1953. In just a few weeks I knew I was in love with Barb. It was getting serious. Mom and Dad liked Barb, but they didn't like the fact that she was a Lutheran. Being a Protestant was bad enough, but a Lutheran! That was the worst!

One thing I particularly liked about Barb was her sense of humor, even if it was at my expense. One night I was scheduled to meet her at the hospital when she got off work at midnight. What I didn't know was that, while I was walking toward the hospital, the police had taken a crazy guy to the emergency room where Barb worked. I learned later that he had asked to go to the men's room and had escaped through the window. He was wearing blue jeans and a white T-shirt. The police rushed out into the streets and fanned out in every direction. Sirens were wailing all around me. I had only a mild curiosity about all the fuss because I was used to hearing sirens in that part of town. I couldn't be bothered with anything except the joy I was feeling about being with Barb in a few minutes. I was on top of the world with absolutely no worries at that moment. Still I wondered what was going on. I found out very soon, because I was walking merrily down the sidewalk, whistling, anticipating being with my girl, wearing blue jeans, and a white T-shirt! Before I knew what had happened, two big policemen grabbed me, one on each side. I said, "Hey, what gives?"

"What's your name, buddy?"

I thought, *Hey, this is a free country. I haven't done anything. Maybe they're kidding.* So I said, "Mickey Mouse."

I knew they weren't kidding when they twisted my arms around behind my back. One policeman yelled to the other officers, "OK, we got him!"

I grimaced in pain, "Hey, you guys, what gives, huh?"

"Take it easy, Mr. Wacko. We'll have you back in the emergency room in just a minute."

What could I do? They wouldn't listen to me. They pushed me through the hospital door, and there stood Barb staring at me. The policeman said, "Is this him, nurse?"

I yelled, "Hey, Barb, tell these guys they caught the wrong man. What is this anyway?"

I watched a mischievous little smile spread over Barb's face as she looked at the policeman and answered, "Yes, that's him."

That little dickens let the charade continue for a few more minutes, and then she confessed to the policemen that I was her boyfriend and she was playing a little joke. Some joke! That's my Barb.

We had a great time together that summer until we had a forced break in our courtship. I had to leave for six weeks of training with the Marines at Quantico, Virginia, in the Platoon Leader Corps. I wasn't too happy about leaving Barb. I experienced some anxieties that maybe our relationship would cool down and eventually go out if we were separated too long. To add to my fears, Barb decided it was time to visit her family in Germany because seven years had passed since she had seen them. So it was with some misgivings that I left for Quantico.

We both got very busy with our own schedules, yet we tried to continue our relationship by mail. But just as I suspected, the letters stopped coming by the end of the summer. I thought it was all over between us. When I came home from Tulsa University for the Christmas holidays in 1953, she was still in Germany. *Maybe she is going to stay there,* I thought. *Maybe her folks have influenced her to break off the relationship.* After all, I was an Italian, and everybody knows that Germans and Italians never got along too well. Even though Barb was of German extraction, she was born in the United States but had spent many years in Germany. I imagined that her family had changed her mind about me and that I would never see her again. I could imagine how they would urge her to stay there because she could get a job as a nurse, especially since she was bilingual. It was going to be a sad Christmas for me.

Christmas passed, but my depression didn't. Not a word from Barb. If she was going to contact me at all, it would be at Christmas, for crying out loud! New Year's Eve came, and I didn't even want to go out. But that night the telephone rang. As soon as I heard that voice on the telephone, my world lit up. It was Barb.

"Sam, my ship just landed in the city. I couldn't contact you because I've been on a tramp steamship for over three weeks. I'm going to the Pallmeyers' in Huntington for a New Year's Eve party. I want you to come. Can you meet me there?"

"Just tell me what time, and I'll be there. Boy, am I glad to hear from you. I love you, Barb."

"I love you, too, Sam."

Floating on air! The whole band was playing again! What a happy New Year's Eve this was. It wasn't over after all. She said she loved me. I didn't waste much time getting started for the Pallmeyers'.

The train from Brooklyn to Huntington seemed to take forever. I just couldn't wait to see Barb. When the train finally arrived, I was the first one off, and she was the first person I saw standing on the platform. For me, it was as if she was the only person there. We rushed to each other and embraced. Clark Gable couldn't have done it any better. Besides, he was only acting; this was real. At the moment I wasn't interested in the party. All I wanted to do was spend the rest of the evening alone with Barb. However, it was a big family gathering and a homecoming for Barb and her sister, Brigitte. We found ourselves struggling all evening to find the time to be alone.

When the Pallmeyers invited me to stay all night, I gladly accepted. After the party ended, we reacquainted ourselves in the family room and, as usual, talked until dawn. It was during this time that we really decided our relationship had stood the test of time. Once again Barb explained how she had been unable to contact me on the tramp steamer. She couldn't call me on the telephone from the ship because she had used all her money to buy her ticket. Only a young person would board ship with just one nickel! Fortunately, the price of the ticket included her meals. The steamer's route was not direct to New York. It stopped at many ports on the way, and that's why the trip took about three weeks. She was worried about it, but there was nothing she could do. I was relieved to learn why she hadn't written or called.

At the Pallmeyers' that weekend, I began to see how strong the spiritual influence was in Barb's life. We were staying in a Protestant minister's parsonage. Sam Rutigliano, Roman Catholic, eating and talking with a Protestant minister. I figured I'd have to go to confession the first chance I got. But I was really impressed with Pastor Pallmeyer and his wife. They were very nice to me; *sweet* is a better word. I wasn't used to seeing such sweet-spirited clergymen. Some of my most fearful moments had come when a priest was chewing me out. The truth is, I probably had it coming! As for seeing a clergyman with a wife, that was just too much. Priests didn't have wives, everybody knew that. It took me a while to stop staring at them. Of course, at that time I didn't understand anything about "the spirit," but I began to see some life qualities in this family that really appealed to me. As a Catholic, I was both wary and curious. I hadn't spent a total of five minutes with a Protestant minister before this in my whole lifetime. They really loved

Barb. I figured if they loved Barb and she loved them, that was good enough for me. I wanted to hang around and find out how these people had gotten to be so nice. This business of love was not new to me because we had a lot of love in our family. But there seemed to be an extra dimension in this family I wanted to know more about. I was full of wonder as this new dimension of love between Barb and me seemed to blossom.

I thought back to the beginning of the summer when Barb and I had been dating heavily. Then I went to the marine camp and she went to Germany. When we parted, we seemed committed to each other. Then four months passed with letters from Barb coming less often and finally, for several weeks, stopping altogether. Now, here we were pledging our love to each other and agreeing to get married in May, just five short months away.

# CHAPTER SEVEN

# LOVE DECLARED

During the Christmas holidays in 1953, Barb and I declared our love for each other. We began discussing marriage on New Year's Eve, and that brought up a subject I had been dreading to face. I had been content to postpone the problem, but the time had come to face it. I had great anxiety about what Mom and Dad would say. I had an absolute fear about what the priest would say. I knew we had gotten to the point in our relationship where these differences had to be dealt with. I would rather have run head-on tackling practice all day than have to face the priest. He would throw everything in the book at me. During all the years I was growing up, I had seen my share of priests laying down the law to people, including me. I didn't quite know what to do. I even thought about the possibility of backing out. But I just couldn't think long about it. Already I hated ever having to leave Barb. And it was time for me to return to Tulsa. I knew then there was no way I was going to break up with this girl. Still I didn't have the courage to open the subject with Mom and Dad yet. So I went back to Tulsa leaving everything hanging. This time, when I left Barb, I hated parting from her more than ever before.

After only about a month passed, I couldn't stand not seeing Barb. It was fifteen hundred miles from Tulsa to New York City, and a plane ticket cost more than I could afford. But I had to see her, and so I flew home in February. We could hardly wait for May to arrive. I still wasn't ready to talk with Mom and Dad and the priest, though. Meantime I returned once again to Tulsa for spring football practice. Barb was on my mind so much I had difficulty concentrating. When Easter arrived, I flew home again, even though my cash position was in desperate shape. I decided it was time to talk to Mom and Dad, but I wasn't so sure about talking to the priest.

When I finally got up my courage, I called Mom and Dad into our kitchen "conference" room where all the family discussions were held and decisions were made. I was troubled about it because I anticipated the worst. I just wanted to get it over with, one way or the other. They would either blow up or tell me to get out of their lives or . . . who knew what they might do. All I knew was that I loved Barb and that I was going to marry her—no matter who said or did what, including the priest. I could still be a Catholic and go to the Catholic church while Barb went to the Lutheran church. Lots of people did that. I mean, what was the big deal? Church is church. The only thing was that nobody in our entire extended family had ever married a non-Italian. More than that, nobody had ever married outside the Catholic church. I was on the brink of committing both sins. I was fearful that Mom and Dad simply couldn't be objective about this kind of thing. Commitment to the idea of Italians marrying Italians within the Catholic church ran deep in our family. I anticipated an emotional scene. When we settled down at the kitchen table, I was nervous but resolved.

"Mom, Dad, I have something important to tell you. Barb and I are going to get married." I wanted to talk fast so they couldn't interrupt me until I got the whole story out. Not daring to look at Dad, I directed my comments to Mom as I spoke, "I know you always expected me to marry a nice Italian-Catholic girl. I always thought I would, too. I know all our relatives expect that, and I also know how everybody is going to be disappointed. I don't even want to talk about what the priest will say. I know what he'll say. I can live with that. I haven't decided yet whether I'll stay in the Catholic church or not. Barb won't leave the Lutheran church, that's for sure. But what I really want is your blessing. You've been terrific parents. I couldn't have asked for better parents. You and Dad have taught me things I'll remember all my life. You've given me values I'll pass on to my children one of these days."

Mom put her hand on my arm and said, "We've known for a long time that you were serious about Barbara. She's a lovely girl. Sure, we hoped you would find someone who was raised like you were, but you and Barbara have found each other. Don't worry about it. As long as you love each other, things will work out. God will be in your corner."

I was caught almost off guard. What a sweetheart Mom was! I was braced for a lot of resistance, maybe even tears. What a mom! I said, "You know, Mom, you're full of love. That's where I've learned all about love, from you." I still hadn't looked at Dad. I expected the worst was yet to come. I looked over at him as he spoke.

"Hey, Sam, it's OK with yer mudda'n me. Barb's a nice goil. We like 'er. So she's not Italian, so——" His voice trailed off as he shrugged. I could hardly believe it. Their reactions were such a relief to me I could almost kiss Dad. In fact I did! But I still wasn't totally off the hook. Mom wanted me to visit the priest, which I agreed to do. Before I left I said, "Look, Mom, Dad, no matter what happens, nothing will ever change between us." We hugged each other, and all three of us had moist eyes. I left the house walking on air.

When I arrived at the priest's office, I was scared but somehow determined. I guess I knew how it would come out. I had never heard of any priest giving his blessing without certain conditions being met. Sure enough, he was plainly pained when I told him I planned to marry a Lutheran. He told me that I could not marry her unless she became a Catholic. He said that if she loved me, she would gladly change. Furthermore, he said I had to sign a contract promising to raise any children Catholic. By the time I left the priest, I was frustrated and confused because I knew when the wedding was announced Mom and Dad would take a lot of flack from our relatives and friends. Barb would be the very first non-Italian in the family and also the first non-Catholic. It was going to be rough, but I was determined to marry Barb—no matter what.

I decided to talk with Pastor Pallmeyer. He said Barb had been raised in a parsonage as a Lutheran. He and his wife had fully expected that Barb would someday marry in the Lutheran church. He was a beautiful, Christian man. I had never been around a person with whom I had been more at home. His advice was that we should pray about it and that God would help us both. He gave no edicts or pronouncements, nor did he impose any conditions.

The final thought I had about marrying Barb was that if we were to have children and they were like she was, that would be good enough for me. That clinched it.

# CHAPTER EIGHT

# THAT'S WHAT HE DESERVES, BUT IT'S NOT WHAT HE NEEDS

**W**ith my new bachelor of arts degree from Tulsa University, I was ready to lick the world in February 1956. Barb and I returned to Brooklyn and moved in with my parents temporarily. I got a job with Commercial Credit Corporation in Hempstead on Long Island, and Barb went to work as a nurse in a hospital. I had almost decided to stay with Commercial Credit when I received a call from Bill Eisenberg, an old friend.

"Hey, Sam, how would you like to be a coach and a teacher?"

"I don't know, but I'd sure like to hear about it."

"I need help on the coaching staff at Midwood High School. How would you like to interview for the job?"

"Tell me more about it, Bill. Does the job include classroom teaching?"

"Well, yes, but not in the usual way."

"What do you mean?"

"I can get you a job teaching, but not at Midwood. I mean, they only need a coach, not a teacher."

"Oh, so it's a part-time coaching job?"

"The coaching at Midwood is part-time, but I can get you set up with a teaching job at George Westinghouse Vocational High School."

"Bill, George Westinghouse is a vocational school in a tough South Brooklyn neighborhood, and Midwood is on the other side of Brooklyn. Midwood is in Flatbush. I'd be traveling all day every day."

"I know, Sam, but it's a start. Wouldn't you like this kind of setup better than collecting delinquent accounts?"

"Actually, I do have my heart set on being a coach, Bill."

So I got the job, that is, both jobs. My first job as a "professional" coach. After all, if I got paid for coaching, even a little, that made me a professional. That job, unimportant as it might seem to some, marked the beginning of my coaching career and had a lasting influence on my life. I'll never forget how proud and excited I was the first day I took the boys out on the practice field. I was almost beside myself when I noticed my dad ambling over to the fence. He had come to watch his son's first day as a coach! I was on top of the world. I watched Dad from the corner of my eye as he leaned on the fence with his hands up high gripping the wire. He didn't come onto the field. He just stood there watching. After a short while, he walked away.

Later that night I dropped by the house. Dad was sitting in the kitchen. I couldn't wait to hear his reaction to seeing me on my first day as a coach. Maybe he would see how a person could make a living out of sports. I hoped he would be proud of me. I walked into the kitchen, beaming, "Hey, Dad, what's happenin'? I saw you watchin' our practice this afternoon. So, what d'ja think, huh?"

He stared at me and said, "Why doncha get a real job?"

That took the wind out of me. Dad just couldn't believe I could make a living by being involved in sports. But a start is a start. Even Vince Lombardi had to start somewhere. Dad only dampened my enthusiasm a short while. I was still excited about coaching.

Teaching at George Westinghouse Vocational High School was another matter. There were many street-tough young men who often reminded me of myself. When I first arrived, the principal received me in his office.

"Well, Sam, welcome to George Westinghouse."

"Thank you. It's good to be here."

"So this will be your first teaching experience since graduating from Tulsa University?"

"Yessir."

"You know, Sam, it's quite different from Tulsa, Oklahoma, here, but I'm sure you know that, having been raised in Brooklyn."

"Yessir, it certainly is different. That's oil and cow country out there. I never saw such wealth."

"That's what I mean. The boys who attend here are not wealthy by any stretch of the imagination. In fact, they're often just a meal or two away from poverty."

"Yessir, I can understand that."

"They talk much differently in Tulsa, too, don't they?"

"Yessir, they sure do." I laughed a little nervously because I suspected he was leading up to something in a roundabout way.

"Sam, these boys are a few of the lucky ones who are brought in off the streets. They'll probably have limited careers and incomes all their lives. At least they have more hope than many others."

"Yessir." I wished he would come to the point, but I was new to this and he was a veteran of one of the toughest school systems in America. I respected him without knowing much about him. Finally, he got to it.

"Sam, you know how street boys talk."

"Yessir." I knew he was referring to the type of language you hear young guys using on every playground and on every street corner.

"Let me ask you something, Sam. What would you do if you were monitoring the study hall or a homeroom class and you heard a lad use *that* four-letter word?"

"I don't know. I never thought about it before."

"Well, think about it, Sam, because you're going to hear it over and over."

"What would you advise me to do if it happens?"

"Not *if*, Sam, *when*. I wouldn't pay much attention to it if I were you."

I thanked him for his advice and began my teaching career. Not too many days passed before I found myself in charge of a homeroom class. One lad in the class caused continual trouble, even on an average day. This particular day he was more surly than usual. I decided to ask him a question. When I heard him mumble something loud enough for only his buddies to hear and snicker their approval for, I felt my blood preparing me for some kind of action. I didn't like surly, mouthy guys, no matter where I found them. I had a problem I had to deal with. My authority was being challenged in front of a bunch of young guys who were watching our every move. The new teacher was going to have his mettle tested. I knew it had to happen sooner or later. It promised to be a shoot-out of some kind at the very least. I walked out from behind my desk, stuck my jaw out, and stared at him.

"What did you say?" I asked.

He jumped up from his seat, stabbed his finger into the air repeatedly, and screamed, "—— you!"

There it was, *the* word. I didn't hesitate. I just reacted. I slugged him and knocked him down in the aisle in front of all his peers. Nobody moved. There was no sound in the classroom. I came to my senses with a jolt. I had struck a student. I'd probably be fired on the spot. Didn't the principal warn me about this? He had gone to great lengths to advise me how to handle such a situation, and I had ignored his advice. I was as wrong as the kid, probably more wrong. I was supposed to know better. Maybe my teaching career would be over before it got off the ground.

I quickly knelt and helped the boy up and into his chair. He was still groggy. When the bell rang, I felt as if I was the one who had been saved by the bell. The class filed silently out. I looked at the boy, and he seemed to be all right. Immediately, I went to the principal's office to "turn myself in." When I told him what had happened, he was upset with me. When he had finished correcting me, he said something I've remembered ever since. "Sam, slugging the boy is what he deserved, but it wasn't what he needed. I'm sure his father will be down here tomorrow. We'd better get ready for him. It could be nasty."

Now I'd done it. On my first teaching job I was already a miserable failure. I imagined all kinds of terrible things that might happen when the boy's father came to the school. I would be called to the principal's office, and the boy's father would be out for blood, my blood. Maybe I didn't want to teach in this school anyway. Maybe I wouldn't have a choice. Hey, maybe the kid's old man would pull a gun or a knife on me. My imagination was working overtime.

Sure enough, the next day I was summoned to the principal's office. "The principal's office." That simple phrase had always carried the threat of doom for me. I didn't like principals' offices. They had always meant trouble for me. It was like saying "the Police Precinct Office." It implied ultimate authority to me, the final appeal in all of life—army, navy, marines, Dad, and the Supreme Court. Funny, I felt almost the same way that day as I walked to the principal's office as a teacher, but still in trouble.

Inside the office, I saw my young tattletale student glaring at me. His father stood beside him. I braced myself. I kept my eyes on his hands. Would he try to slug me? Would he reach into his pockets for whatever weapon he might have hidden? I stayed near the door. My track experience might come in handy in a minute or two. This guy could never catch me. Who wants to be a teacher anyway?

The principal introduced the boy's father to me. I held out my hand. To my amazement, he took my hand and shook it.

Then he turned to his son. "See dis man here, son? He's a teacher, see? When you're at dis school, he's da boss, see? You do what he says, see? If you don't I'll give you more to worry about dan he has, see?"

I breathed a sigh of relief. It could have been much different. I was lucky. Today, at this writing, I would have been hauled into court and sued for my actions. I'm certain that I could not survive as a full-time career teacher in today's classrooms.

That was the first of many lessons I was to learn as a teacher: reward in public, censure in private. As I left school that evening, I kept recalling the principal's words: "Slugging the boy is what he deserved, but it wasn't what he needed."

My teaching career had been launched, but it hadn't been easy. Where would it lead me? What would happen next in my life? I didn't think of asking God for help, for I didn't know who or where He was. But I had the confidence of youth. I was going to be a coach, a successful coach. I was a jock, a good jock. Word would get out all over the school about how I clobbered that mouthy kid. Maybe the boys wouldn't like me, but they would respect me. The teachers would probably give me a medal. With the safe passage of the scene in the principal's office, I gained new confidence in myself. Maybe I could handle this teaching career after all. It proved to be much easier to handle than the next chapter in my life.

# CHAPTER NINE

# TOUGH TIMES, HIGH TIMES WITH GOD

Our little Nancy lived only four and a half years. She was close to God from the very beginning of her life. She loved to laugh and have fun. She had a warmth about her that evoked involuntary smiles and spontaneous hugs, even from strangers. She had dark hair, sparkling brown eyes, light skin, and a sense of humor that was both innocent and well-developed.

Once when we were all at a summer camp dinner table, sitting there with the owners of the camp and many others all around, Nancy looked at me and said without warning, for all the world to hear, "Now, Dad, please don't expel gas at the dinner table." Where that came from no one knows. She was serious but humorous, innocent but knowing. Everyone roared with laughter, which gave me time to recover from my embarrassment. I was aghast, no pun intended.

It was back in 1962 when Barb, Nancy, and I were visiting my brother in Montreal, Canada. We left his home at midnight in order to arrive back in Maine the next morning where Barb and I were on the staff of a summer camp. I was the athletic director, and Barb was the camp nurse. She had to return in time to give some of the kids their medication. The still, clear night gave no hint of the terror that was coming.

I had removed the rear seat of our Volkswagen so Nancy could sleep back there. We drove a long time and then stopped for doughnuts and coffee. Daylight was just breaking when we climbed back in the VW. Nancy was so tired and sleepy that she began to whimper. I gave her a doughnut to settle her down, and after a while I looked back to see if she was asleep. That's the last thing I remember inside the car. When I regained consciousness, I was sitting on an asphalt road in front of a farmhouse. I had fallen asleep at the wheel. Apparently the VW rolled all the way over and came to rest on its wheels on the pavement.

As if awakening from a deep sleep, I focused my eyes on the asphalt pavement. Where was I? Groggy and confused, I wondered why I was sitting in the middle of an asphalt road. My rib cage felt blazing hot. My hands were blistered and bloody. I looked around and saw the Volkswagen sitting where it had landed upright on its wheels. Then, a horrible paralysis seized me while I looked around at the unreal world about me. I'm sure I froze for only a few seconds, but it seemed that time had stopped and I hung suspended in a scene from a nightmare. Surely I would awaken and all this unbelievable horror would dissolve.

Still disoriented, I heard the echoes of shattering glass and crunching metal in my mind. *My God, what about Barb and Nancy?* I jumped up and felt a searing pain in my side. I saw Barb still sitting in the front passenger seat, dazed and covered with her own blood. I lunged toward the VW and pulled Barb out of the seat. Then I looked in the backseat for Nancy. She wasn't there.

*Nancy, Nancy, my God, where is my little Nancy?* I ran to the back of the VW, and my breath was choked off as if I had run into an unseen clothesline. *Oh, God!* I saw her under the wheel. No movement in her little body. She was as limp and lifeless as a broken doll. I sucked in air as I stared death in the face. No one had to tell me. She was dead. Barb screamed and knelt beside her, oblivious to her own bloody wounds, and gave her mouth-to-mouth resuscitation. Nancy was not breathing.

People poured out of the farmhouse, saw what had happened, and someone ran to call an ambulance. Twenty-five long minutes passed before help arrived. I stood there numb as the doctor looked up at me from where he was kneeling beside Nancy. I already knew what he was going to say, yet the finality of the official pronouncement swept away any lingering thread of hope. "She's gone," he said.

They took Barb and me to a hospital in Berlin, New Hampshire, where we were treated in the emergency room and then admitted to a room together in the hospital. It was to be the toughest twenty-four hours we ever spent together. Barb cried all day and night. Neither of us slept. Anguish, guilt, and despair pounded our thoughts: *How can we go on? How could this happen? How could God bring someone like Nancy into the world and then allow her to be killed so violently? How? Why?* All night long we lay there crying and questioning. We had broken ribs and lacerations, but it was our minds and hearts that had been devastated.

Even though Barb was completely filled with grief, she did something right after her release from the hospital that still astounds me when I recall it. She insisted on returning to the summer camp long enough to administer medications to the various children in her charge. What a tremendous sense of responsibility she had. After that, we drove to Huntington, Long Island, to meet my parents who were bringing our son, Paul, to meet us. Paul still did not know that his little sister was dead. We faced the ordeal of telling him.

When my parents drove up and I watched Paul get out of the car, I was overcome with emotion. To see our remaining child alive caused a tidal wave of gratitude to sweep through my body. Barb cried, and we both hugged him close. I stood there watching him, wondering what it was going to be like with only one child and how Paul would take it. For four and a half of his seven years, he had played constantly with his little sister. Now we would all miss her on birthdays and Christmases and summers and trips.

Not only did I wonder how Paul was going to cope with it, I kept wondering the same about Barb and me. Even if we had another baby next year, Paul would be eight years older than any new child and probably too old to play with him or her. It would be like having two families. On the other hand, if we had no additional children, Paul was it. Nancy was gone. I had to face it, and I had to cause Paul to understand, too.

All those thoughts came into my mind, and I didn't want them there. I was almost angry with myself for the train of thought that had thundered into my mind. I just couldn't cope with it. All I could think of was how to tell Paul about Nancy. It wasn't a question of getting through a day at a time; it was a question of getting through an hour at a time.

While family and close friends gathered around to give us sympathy, I focused on the fact that Paul was alive. What had caused us not to take him on the trip with us? The question haunted me. Barb could hardly speak at all. For the moment, all we could do was hug Paul and thank God he was spared. When he asked where Nancy was, I held him close. The time had come. I put him down and said, "Let's go for a walk, Paul."

He repeated his question, "Where's Nancy, Daddy?"

I cleared my throat and hesitated for a moment. I just couldn't bring myself to tell him she had been killed. I shuddered as the accident scene forced itself into my mind with all its fresh horror. I cleared my throat again. Then, close to tears myself, I said quietly, "Paul, Nancy is no longer here. She's gone to heaven."

"What do you mean, Daddy? Where is she?"

"Paul, she's gone to be with God." Isn't that what parents are supposed to say in situations like this? I didn't know what to say. I didn't know God. Why was I telling Paul that? That's all I could think of to say. I knew he would be at the funeral and we would have to go through a lot of grief together. It was going to be tough for him to let go of his little sister. But first it was going to be tough for him to understand that she was dead. His questions came in bursts.

"Why is she gone? Why did she go to heaven? Why can't I see her now? Won't I ever see her again?"

"God wants her to be with Him."

"Why, Daddy?"

I knew I couldn't answer Paul's question because I had the same question in my mind. Mine was a lame attempt to answer my son's question. I didn't know how he accepted it. I couldn't probe that seven-year-old mind.

"Daddy, will Nancy still sleep in her room?"

"No, honey."

"Will she be able to watch cartoons with me?"

"No, honey."

Somehow we got through the next few days one day at a time. Barb's pain was so great that she simply sat around the house, crying. I had to eventually return to work, but it wasn't easy. The funeral was still to come.

# CHAPTER TEN

# FEAR KNOCKED AT THE DOOR, FAITH ANSWERED

**N**ancy's funeral was in August of 1962 at the Lutheran church in Greenwich, Connecticut. Barb and I decided we didn't want to have a wake. I had seen so many of them as I grew up. In Italian families they often last for three days. We just couldn't face up to that. Knapp Funeral Home handled the closed-casket funeral with only the immediate family in attendance at the funeral home. Just before her death, Nancy had been begging Barb for some new clothespins to use as she played house. Barb had never bought them, and she was distressed over it. She checked with stores all over town until she found some clothespins. It tore my heart out to see my wife putting those clothespins in Nancy's casket. Pastor Henry Heck officiated at the funeral and really ministered to Barb and me.

The day of the funeral we were still struggling with the question of why such a thing could happen to a four-and-a-half-year-old girl. We could not say, "Thy will be done." We wanted to know why it had happened. We went to the church, and many of the young boys I had coached in New York City and at Greenwich were there. The church was right across the street from the high school and the athletic field. I had been there from 1959 to 1961, running back and forth on the athletic field, always just across from the church. Now I was at the church looking across at the school and the athletic field, wondering at how different everything was then. Barb had always brought Nancy and Paul to our games there. Who would have thought Nancy would be lying in a casket in that church before she reached five years of age? I couldn't sort it all out as I sat there in the church. Pastor Heck gave a marvelous service with a beautiful sermon. He quoted the Scripture that promised, "In My Father's house are many mansions; . . . I go to prepare a place for you." Although it was comforting, I still felt a tremendous emptiness and void. I had no idea how Barb and I were going to be able to reconstruct our lives. After the eulogy, we walked to the door of the church. We knew some of the people weren't going to the cemetery so we wanted to thank them for coming before they left the church.

As we worked our way back through the crowd of people toward the door, George and Jean Schwamb, two Christian friends who belonged to the church, came up to comfort us. They had lost their son, George, Junior, who had drowned a few years earlier when he was eight years old. They tried to minister to us, but we were just not listening well. We couldn't fathom why this had happened to us. But George gently grabbed both Barb and me and spoke these words, "Barb, Sam, this will be one of the most glorious days of your life if you will accept Jesus Christ. If you ask Him to enter into your lives right now and simply say, 'Thy will be done,' He will begin to fill that void and emptiness you feel now. He will begin to give you the wisdom, the knowledge, the hope, the character, and the perseverance to be able to cope with this tragedy."

For a few seconds I considered pushing him aside. Everybody else who spoke with us showed pity and compassion, but this man was telling us something so drastically different that I was confused and perplexed at first. I was tempted to be very angry with him. How insensitive can you get? Couldn't he see we were still crying?

I searched his eyes. There was no hint of sarcasm or cynicism. I saw nothing but compassion and warmth. His eyes held mine as if I was suspended in space while time stood still. Eternity had somehow closed in around me. In my mind's eye I was in a tunnel on a highway approaching a curve I couldn't see around. My resistance began to crumble as I sensed the importance of what was occurring. I was passing around the curve on the road in my mind. I began to see a faint light of hope ahead. The light grew brighter as I approached the end of the tunnel. I felt at last that help was there.

This was what I had heard about and avoided all my life. People who talked the way my friend was talking had always turned me off. But I suddenly saw the spiritual poverty of my life. I had been in a dark place, full of self, of ambition, of scratching to win and have things my way. I had already accepted a huge burden of guilt for falling asleep in the car. Already I blamed myself for Nancy's death. I couldn't bring Nancy back to life. I didn't know if I could bear up under this burden in the future. I desperately needed help at that moment in suspended time. I didn't realize how desperately I needed it until I heard my friend's words. I understood at last that this Jesus, whom I had heard about all my life, whose name I had used in vain, was my only source of help. I began to catch vague glimpses of how much He must love us, for He was reaching out to me at that very moment. I neither saw nor heard anything except this man. Something of monumental importance was happening. It was as if I were drowning and thrashing around in the water somewhere while someone was asking me if I would be willing to ask for a life preserver.

Then suddenly a peace that passed understanding seemed to envelope me. I began to listen to this man, hearing him for the first time. Wait a minute! These people really did know how we felt. They had lost a child, too. This was no weird joke. I knew I wanted to pray with them more than anything else in the world at that moment. Eagerly I said, "Yes, Lord Jesus, come into my life." Barb did, too. The Schwambs hugged us and cried along with us.

When we got to the cemetery, it was a beautiful sunny day. Nancy's grave site was next to a fence that surrounded a school yard full of playground equipment. She would have liked to be near the playground. Maybe the location of her grave contributed to my feelings, but I felt a sereneness I had never experienced before. Nancy was with the Lord, safe for eternity. Now we had met Him. Now we would be on the same page with Him.

As we walked away from the grave site, the Schwambs walked with us. Both Barb and I talked about the new serenity we felt. I said to George and Jean, "This sense of peace is a strange new feeling for us. We want to thank you both for what you've done."

"Sam, Jean and I know exactly what you mean. Being here with you and Barb has helped us tremendously because we haven't felt the presence of the Lord so strongly since we lost little George."

Slowly, as silent and gentle as descending mist at evening, I felt a covering from above, a surrender, a willingness to say, for the first time, "Thy will be done." It had happened. The peace that passes understanding. So that's how it felt and what it meant.

We drove back to New York City and spent some time with my family. They found it difficult to understand our serenity. All their prior experience with death and wakes was associated with much crying and wailing. As days passed, I was still often tempted to become angry or upset, but each time I was able to say, "Thy will be done." God always gave me the strength I needed to keep going. He was always there by my side.

Meantime, I had to go back to work, and we had to get on with our lives. I was starting a new job at Horace Greeley High School in Chappaqua, New York. I had to rent out our home in Bethel, Connecticut, and get established in Greenwich, Connecticut. It was important for us to be close to the Schwambs and Pastor Heck, who lived in Greenwich. They and our neighbors, Martha and Ed Chiappetta, ministered to us. All of them were tremendous sources of encouragement at that time in our lives. There were moments of real loneliness and depression during that first year following Nancy's death. As each holiday or birthday rolled around, it brought fresh and painful memories of Nancy. Our friends were always there when we needed them. They would drag us out of the house to go for a pizza or to a movie. They shared many hours of dialogue with us. They were real gifts from God. Pastor Heck was really God's representative to us. We were brand-new Christians needing the fellowship and follow-up necessary to help us grow spiritually. He provided that help. The entire church family, led by Pastor Heck, surrounded us with love and support. They helped us answer many questions and also to accept the fact some questions are unanswerable in this life.

Many times as I drove home from work at night, I would anticipate the scene at home. Then it would hit me afresh that Nancy wouldn't be there. I would feel almost overwhelmed with grief, and I would pull the car over to the side of the road and pray. For the first few months after Nancy's death, Barb was devastated. She couldn't bring herself to cook or have any interest in doing anything. She wanted to be alone with me and not anybody else, not even family. She just wanted to suffer out her grief. Barb's parents came from Germany to visit, but Barb couldn't handle having any visitors, and they didn't stay long.

To add to this terrible tragedy, something else happened—Barb had become pregnant. In her ninth month, she went to the hospital. I stayed with her awhile, but the baby didn't come. I went home and was awakened at about five in the morning by the telephone. The nurse said, "Mr. Rutigliano, we think you'd better come to the hospital right away."

"What's wrong?" My knees went weak. "Is Barb all right?"

"Yes, she's all right, but why don't you come on down and we'll talk to you then."

I rushed to the hospital, praying and worrying, wondering what else could possibly happen to us. When I arrived, they told me that Barb had had a stillborn baby girl. It was almost too much for us to bear. I stayed at the hospital with Barb for the next three days until I could take her home. We didn't know what to think or what to do. Maybe we just weren't supposed to have more children. Paul, in the meantime, stayed with neighbors.

After a period of recovery for Barb, we decided to look into the adoption process. We talked to an agency in New York City and to friends who had adopted children. The agency assured us they could match us with an Italian-and-German parental lineage. We filled out all the papers and were close to finalizing the agreement when we discovered that Barb was pregnant. God was with us. Alison and Kerry were born in Greenwich in 1964 and 1967.

So we had learned a great deal about birth and death. But most important, we had learned about being born again.

# CHAPTER ELEVEN

# THE PRICE IS NOT RIGHT

I coached at the high-school level from 1956 to 1964 working at such schools as Lafayette High School in Brooklyn, New York, Horace Greeley High School in Chappaqua, New York, and Greenwich High School in Greenwich, Connecticut. But then something happened that would take me out of the high schools and into college coaching.

In June 1964 I was invited to interview for an assistant coach's job at the University of Connecticut. I was flattered because I knew what an outstanding staff they had—Lou Holtz from Kent State who, at this writing (you never know in the coaching profession!), is head coach at Notre Dame; Rick Forzano from Kent State, who became head coach for Navy and also was the head coach of the Detroit Lions; Dave Adolph from the University of Akron, who is now defensive coordinator for the Cleveland Browns; and Dan Sekanovich, who is now defensive line coach for the Miami Dolphins. How could I fit into such a great group?

I broke the news to Barb, "Honey, I've been invited to interview for a job at the University of Connecticut."

"I thought you were going to stay at the high-school level. You've said yourself that once you make that move from high school to college, it'll never be the same. This is a lifetime job here."

"I know."

"If you move to college, the next move will be to the pros, and we'll probably move every three years."

I said, "Look, I don't think I have a chance of getting the job, but it would be a nice little drive for us. I'll probably finish the interview by the middle of the morning, and we can have a nice lunch and then drive home." So we drove to the campus and I left Barb in the student union building.

Rick Forzano, the head coach, was gracious, but he didn't seem overly enthusiastic about my being there. As the interview progressed, however, he seemed to take on new interest. Then he asked each member of the coaching staff to interview me. The middle of the morning came and went. By the time all the men had talked to me, it was lunchtime. Rick invited me to go to lunch at the student union cafeteria. I decided not to tell them that Barb was waiting for me. I sensed that they were about to offer me a job, and I didn't want them to feel rushed. When we went into the cafeteria, I spotted Barb sitting alone at a table. She looked at me, but I didn't acknowledge her presence in any way. We finished our lunch and walked toward the door. I didn't so much as wink at her. For a few seconds I thought the steam I saw from her coffee had risen from her nostrils! I just walked out as if she didn't exist.

When we got back to Rick's office in the gym, he wanted to keep talking. We talked until 6:00 P.M.! I had no idea where Barb was or when the student union closed. Well, she had the car to wait in, right? Just when I thought we were finished, Rick asked, "How would you like to play racketball?"

I said, "Sure, why not?"

Finally, at 8:00 P.M., after I showered and said good-bye to Rick, I sprinted over to the student union. Barb was nowhere to be seen. I walked out to the parking lot where I had parked the car twelve hours earlier. No car, no Barb. After looking around, I found the car in another parking place. The windows were so steamed up I couldn't see inside—boy, was she mad. I opened the door and slid nonchalantly into the driver's seat. Barb looked straight ahead. With my opening remark, I knew I was dead meat! I tried to explain the situation, but I got nowhere with her. There was no reasoning with her. We drove all the way back with me, Professor Harold Hill of *The Music Man*, doing all the talking. She never said a word. To this day she gets mad when we talk about it. It was one of the dumbest things I ever did in my life. After having spent all that time, I still hadn't been offered the job. I had to tell Barb that Rick was going to call me to let me know.

Somehow, Rick found out that Barb had waited for me all that time and that I had been unwilling to tell him. He called me and said, "Sam, anybody who wants this job bad enough to risk his neck with his wife can have it. You've got the job if you still want it." And so we went to the University of Connecticut.

In 1964 we had a good year, but 1965 was superexciting. We beat Yale in our opener that year. You have to understand how significant that statement is. For the first time in eighty-five years, a Connecticut team beat Yale University; that was *our* team! The rest of that season was anticlimactic. By the end of the season, I was already becoming impatient to get to a higher college sports level. I was really looking forward to the coaches' convention that year because that's where coaches meet and recruit each other.

The entire University of Connecticut assistant coaching staff drove together from Storrs, Connecticut, to Washington, D.C., to attend the American Football Coaches' Association Convention at the Shoreham Hotel. In the car were Lou Holtz, Dan Sekanovich, Dave Adolph, and I. There would be thousands of coaches attending the convention, most with the same agenda: to find a better job with a bigger school. Everybody wanted to get acquainted with the great coaches from the top colleges with great traditions and great locations.

Lou Saban had just left the Buffalo Bills after being elected 1964 and 1965 Coach of the Year and winning the American Football League Championship in both 1964 and 1965. His resignation from the Bills and appearance as head coach at the University of Maryland had everyone buzzing and wanting to seek him out. He would be hiring a staff, and everybody knew it. Coaches from all over the United States were jockeying for positions, trying to meet with and talk to Lou.

As for myself, I had dreamed about coaching at Maryland. They had been national champions. Maryland was located in the East, close to my home. The university's recruiting activity was done in Pennsylvania, North and South Jersey, Long Island, New York City, Connecticut, and Boston—all the areas in which I had strong recruiting experience. I knew how great it would be if I could get a job with Maryland. Just to have a chance to talk to Lou Saban would be exciting. I fantasized about how the conversation would go. But I didn't have to fantasize long, because I saw him in the hotel lobby the very first day of the convention with what seemed like hundreds of coaches surrounding him. I wended my way toward him and finally stood face-to-face with him.

I thrust out my right hand and said, "Hi, Lou, I'm Sam Rutigliano, on the coaching staff at University of Connecticut."

"Nice to meet you, Sam. I won't try to pronounce your last name."

I laughed and took a deep breath. "Lou, I'd love to have an appointment with you while you're here. I know you're gonna need a staff——"

"Gee, Sam, we've got that pretty well lined up and——"

"I'd really appreciate it if you'd give me just fifteen minutes in the privacy of your room. I mean, it's a madhouse here in the lobby."

"Yeah, well, my schedule is pretty full already. Seems like every coach in America wants to talk to me."

"I can appreciate that. Say, instead of taking any more of your time here, how about scheduling me for just fifteen minutes at 10:00 tomorrow morning? If I can't interest you in that period of time, I'll leave."

"Sam, we've pretty much filled all the positions already and ——"

"Hey, just to be able to talk with you for those few minutes would be the high point of the convention for me. I know it's just one chance in a million, but I'd love to do it if you will."

"Well, all right, I guess we can find fifteen minutes. Ah, what'd you say your name was again?"

"Sam."

"No, I mean your last name?"

"Rutigliano."

"Rutigliano, yeah, OK."

"Just call me Sam. I'll see you tomorrow morning. Thanks, Lou."

I couldn't believe it. Lou Saban had consented to an interview with me! The AFL Coach of the Year was going to talk to me, a guy who had been a high-school coach just two years ago! What a thrill!

That night I walked into the elevator of the hotel and there stood my friend, Dick MacPherson. Little did I know then that one day I would hire Dick as my linebacker coach for the Cleveland Browns and that he would go on to be the head coach for Syracuse University. Dick and I were good friends, and he looked as if he had just won a sweepstakes. I said, "Dick, what's happening?"

"Sam, I'm walking on air. I just accepted a job as linebacker coach for Lou Saban at the University of Maryland. Man, I'm excited."

"Hey, congratulations, Dick! That's terrific. Let me tell you something else exciting. I'm scheduled to talk with Lou tomorrow about a coaching job."

"No kidding? Hey, that's great. I know he's got one more position to fill, but I think he's got the guy he wants. One of the big alums is putting a lot of pressure on Lou to hire this guy who's also a Maryland graduate. Looks like it's all set."

"Well, anyway, I'm gonna talk to Lou tomorrow. Anything you can do to help, I'd really appreciate."

"I'll sure keep it in mind, Sam. Good luck tomorrow."

"Thanks, Dick. I'll see you later."

I sat around until about 3:00 A.M. talking to the guys, sharing hopes and dreams, until I had to get to bed. I was too excited to sleep much anyway and could hardly wait for the time for my interview.

When I arrived in the hallway outside Lou's room, it looked like a doctor's waiting room. The hallway was filled with guys waiting to talk to Lou. I took my place in line and stood there for an hour and a half. All the time I was thinking, *I don't have a chance at this job. I'm wasting my time. I might as well go down to the lobby and relax with some friends.* But as I stood there, I rehearsed what I would say and decided to give it my best shot. What would it hurt? It would be a good contact for me at least, and maybe somewhere down the line it would pay off. When my name was called, I went in, but I had only about ten minutes with him. I felt that it was all over for me.

Later that day I ran into Dick MacPherson who said, "Hey, Sam, let me tell you what happened with the guy Saban almost hired."

"Almost hired? You mean the guy didn't get the job?"

"Not yet anyway. Lou interviewed the guy and then told me the guy seemed too self-centered. Lou said he used the pronoun *I* too much. He just didn't like him."

"Hey, you mean I'm still alive?"

"Well, I was in the office a little while ago and saw a long list of names Lou was sending thank-you notes to. Your name was on the list. So I told Lou that I knew you, and he took your name off the list of rejects. I don't know if that means he'll call you, but at least he took your name off the list."

"That's very nice of you, Dick. Thanks very much."

"Hey look, if no other name pops up, he may call you. Hang in there."

That night a bunch of us went out for dinner, and once again we stayed up until about three o'clock. I told myself I wouldn't hear from Lou Saban, but I was still too excited to sleep. I went to bed wondering what the odds were that Lou would call me. I thought, *Maybe he'll call or have someone else call and at least tell me thanks but no thanks.* I did get to meet him and have an interview after all. It would be good experience for the future. Not that many coaches got to talk to Lou during the convention.

At about seven o'clock that morning, the telephone rang. I picked it up and said, "Hello."

"Good morning, Sam. This is Lou Saban."

I thought it must be a joke. Maybe one of my buddies was pulling my leg. I almost said something sarcastic, but fortunately I didn't. Suddenly I realized it really was Lou Saban. "Oh, Lou, how are you?"

"Did I wake you?"

"Oh, no. I've been up a long time."

"Sam, could you have breakfast with me?"

Could I have breakfast with him? Could I have breakfast with Lou Saban?! "Sure! Where? When?"

We made a date to meet in the hotel, and I was so excited I almost didn't hear where he said to meet. I never showered and shaved so fast in my life. I remembered the mistake the other guy made in saying *I* so much. I resolved not to use that pronoun at all if I could avoid it. In record time I was sitting opposite this famous coach and eating breakfast with him. I tried not to be aggressive. I tried my very best not to say *I*. We talked about a lot of things but nothing specific. He was weighing me, testing, using whatever experience he had in sizing up men. All I could think of was to avoid saying *I*. I was getting discouraged about the way things were going. At about 9:30, Lou told me to wait in my room for his call.

I went up to my room feeling mighty low. I sat by that telephone and stared at it. Then I got up and paced the floor, stopping to look out the window with every lap around the room. I couldn't believe that I was even being considered for such a job. My emotions bounced from despair to euphoria and back again.

At one o'clock the phone rang. I jumped up and almost ran to pick it up. "Hello."

"Hi, Sam. Lou Saban here. Can you stop down at my room in a few minutes?"

"I'll be right there." I hung up the phone and almost did a cartwheel. I said out loud, "Can you believe this?" Within a couple of minutes I was out the door, headed for Lou's room.

Inside the room Lou smiled and said, "I'd like you to join the staff at Maryland, Sam. Congratulations."

"Thank you. I'm honored."

"Now, how'd you say you pronounced that last name of yours?"

"Just call me Sam." We both laughed.

When I left Lou, I went to my room and called Barb. When I told her the good news, she was very excited. We talked and laughed and celebrated on the telephone until finally Barb asked me a question.

"Sam, what will your salary be?"

"What?"

"How much are they going to pay you?"

"Barb, can you believe this? I never even asked."

# CHAPTER TWELVE

# HIRED TO BE FIRED

My entrance into the ranks of professional football came about in an unusual way. I had never entertained any serious thoughts of becoming a coach in the pros. I simply saw myself as a college coach. The entire college scene appealed to me. I was interested in education and character building for young men. My father had indelibly impressed me with the importance of education. To me, football helped in many ways to accomplish this. I had watched young boys become men and young men become better men because of what they learned in football. Suddenly I was faced with a decision for which I was not prepared.

Something strange and exciting happened about two hours before the kickoff of Maryland's last game of the 1966 season. We were in Tallahassee, Florida, matched up against Florida State. I was still assistant coach under Lou Saban. It had been a good season, and we almost won the Atlantic Coast Conference during Lou's first year as coach. There was no way I could have known then that I would be considered for the head coaching job at Maryland in both 1982 and 1986. Coaching, like politics, makes strange bedfellows.

We walked out of the hotel ready to board the bus to take us to the stadium. Lou grabbed me by the arm and said, "Sam, I want to tell you something in the strictest confidence. I've been offered a ten-year contract as head coach and general manager of the Denver Broncos."

"Holy mackerel, Lou! A ten-year contract in the pros?"

"Yep. Ten-year contract."

"But, Lou, not too long ago you said you'd never go back to the pros."

"Yeah, so I changed my mind."

"Hey, I just joined your staff nine months ago, and now you're gonna leave me? What's gonna happen to me? What's gonna happen to the football program at Maryland? Who's gonna take over?''

"Sam, I want you to go with me. The reason you mustn't say anything to any of the other coaches is because I'm not inviting everybody on the staff to go with me."

"Yes, Lou. I'd love to go." Then I remembered that Barb had just had new carpeting installed in our new house. We had been in it only nine months. I grinned at Lou and said, "But I'll take the job only on one condition."

He snapped his head around and stared at me, "What's that?"

"*You* have to tell Barb!"

I got on the bus bursting with excitement, but I couldn't talk about it to anyone, especially anyone on that bus. I wondered why Lou hadn't waited until after the game to tell me. It was going to be difficult to concentrate on the game ahead of us with all that was going through my mind.

The first half was like a dream. We were down by one touchdown when we went into the locker room. We gave the guys the adjustments and a pep talk and went back out to the field for the second half. I went up to the press box and put the headset on so I could talk to Lou, who was on the field. Lou was probably the most impetuous man I ever met. I had no idea how impetuous he was until I heard his voice coming through the earphones.

"Sam, put the headphones down, get yourself a Coke and a hot dog. We're going to Denver."

I spent the next half letting all this sink into my head. I wasn't going to be a coach at Maryland any longer. Lou wasn't wasting any time. I wanted to do my best during that last game for Maryland, but it wasn't easy. We lost the game, and it's no wonder.

After we returned to the Maryland campus Saturday night, I went straight home to tell Barb the "good" news. She met me at the door with a message most coaches have heard from their wives many times.

"Sorry you lost, Sam."

"Barb, you'd better sit down. I have something important to tell you. I have some good news and some bad news."

Barb's eyes darkened as if I had slapped her. "Now what?"

"The bad news is that Lou Saban is resigning tomorrow."

"You mean you don't have a job?"

"I have a job, but it's in Denver, with the Broncos. Lou has a ten-year contract with them, and he wants us to go with him."

She jumped up, "I can't believe this! We've already moved twice this year. I can't believe that you're asking me to sell this house, which we've been in only nine months, and buy a third one—all in the same year. What I *really* can't believe is that you want me to go all the way out to Colorado, which is at the other end of the world."

"Barb, this is the opportunity of a lifetime. I never dreamed that I would have a chance to coach in pro football."

"I told you when you left the high-school coaching job that this would happen. I *don't* want to move. How about the kids? Another school for them? And what about the new baby I'm supposed to have in about thirty days by cesarean section? And the carpet! What about the new carpet? We just ordered it, just made a down payment. Oh, Sam, how could you *possibly* do something like this to me?"

The situation called for all the conning abilities of a Professor Harold Hill, the ultimate con man. Somehow I had to talk Barb into moving again. Although she balked and complained, she finally understood that the career opportunity was surely going to be best for the family in the long run. I knew as well as anyone how difficult coaching changes were for families. It was part of the territory. But for Barb, it was even more difficult. She had grown up in the little village of Steinbach, near Dresden, in Germany, and had always aspired to own a small white house with a white picket fence and live happily ever after. How could she live happily ever after if we moved three times every year? It eventually dawned on both of us that we had, for better or for worse, entered the passing lane of life and there would be no turning back.

On Monday morning, at nine o'clock, I arrived at the University of Maryland and looked for Lou Saban. I found him cleaning out his office in the gym. While I helped him load his station wagon, he said to me, "Sam, you've got a job with me in Denver. Turn in your resignation to the university right away and go home and wait for my phone call." Before I knew what had happened, Lou was out the door and gone, bag and baggage, by 10:00 A.M.

Like a dutiful son, I resigned my job and went home. I looked at Barb and shrugged, "I quit my job."

"Terrific. Don't you think it would have been better to wait a day or two first? How many days can we go without grocery money, waiting for Lou Saban to call?"

"He'll call."

The rest of Monday went by. Barb said, "So why hasn't Lou called?"

"He'll call."

Tuesday came and went. I got nervous.

Barb said, "I'm getting more and more nervous, Sam."

"Don't be nervous, Barb. He said to be ready at a moment's notice."

"I'd settle for any kind of notice. It's not nice to make pregnant ladies nervous, Sam."

"He'll call."

Wednesday arrived. I considered the possibility that Lou had forgotten all about me. *I mean, Lou was impetuous, but he couldn't forget about his assistant coach, could he?* I asked myself. *He'll be calling any second now to tell me to fly to Denver.*

Finally Lou called, "Sam, I want you to get an airline ticket and fly to Miami, get a room at the Everglades Hotel, and go to the North-South College All-Star Game and scout the players." Then he hung up the phone. So I was officially working as a professional football coach. Somehow I didn't feel any different. Of course, all that would change later.

I followed Lou's orders and arrived in Miami with a grand total of ten dollars in my pocket. I called Lou and said, "I'm here in Miami, but I've got only ten bucks cash."

"No problem. I've already called Al Davis. He's staying in the same hotel you're in. It's all set for him to loan you five hundred dollars. Call him." There I was, arriving in the big time, and I didn't have enough money to buy my meals for one day. It seemed too embarrassing for me to go to Al and borrow that money. I needn't have feared, because Al was very gracious and understanding.

After scouting the game and filing my report with Lou, I returned to College Park, Maryland. Plenty of problems awaited me at home. Barb had decided to go back to Connecticut to have the baby because she wanted to use the same doctor she had before. I called Lou and told him about my problems, which included the new baby and the need to sell our house. He was very thoughtful and simply told me to take whatever time was necessary to finalize everything before coming to Denver. I've always appreciated how he treated Barb and me during that time.

The Denver staff was hired, and all had reported to Denver by the end of January 1967—all, that is, except me. Our entire family went to Barb's sister's house in Connecticut to stay there until Barb delivered. On January 13, Kerry was born by cesarean section at Greenwich Hospital in Connecticut. When Barb was able to travel, we drove back to Maryland.

Early in March, we sold our house and flew to Denver. The moving truck would take about seven days to reach Denver. In the meantime we had to locate a house before the truck arrived.

As we approached Denver, Barb said, "Oh, look at the mountains! It reminds me of the Alps."

I said, in my best schoolteacher tone, "Those are the Rockies, Barb."

"I know they're the Rockies, Sam."

We had lots of clever dialogue like that on the trip.

In our hotel room after dinner, I flipped on the television set. We heard an announcer saying something that snapped us all to attention: "The Denver Broncos will probably move to Phoenix, Winston-Salem, or some other city."

I jumped to my feet, "What?!"

Barb simply said, "Terrific. We just get here, and they're leaving. It's like two ships passing in the night."

Profoundly I said, "I can't believe it!"

Barb said, "Our furniture will be here in five or six days, we're living in a hotel like a bunch of gypsies, we don't even have a house to rent, and the Broncos are leaving. I love it!"

"Barb, don't worry. Things'll be all right."

"We'll probably have to store our furniture and live in the car."

"Come on, Barb, don't be silly."

"I wonder if Lou still has a job? Ugh, coaching!"

"Hey, don't worry, he's got a ten-year contract."

"Sam, according to this announcer, the team may end up anywhere in the United States. Welcome to Denver, Rutiglianos."

"Hey, don't sweat it, Barb. That's probably just hype to get the Denver fans to commit to an advance season-ticket sale. Everything's gonna be OK. I'll call Lou first thing in the morning. Hey, with all your real estate experience, you'll have us a house in a jiffy."

"How and where am I going to find us a house?"

"Hey, Barb, you're terrific. I know you. You'll have a great house for us in no time." I mean, what is a coach's wife for, right? Besides, she had personally bought and sold more homes than some real estate sales persons, and she's never had a license! The problem was finally resolved when we rented a four-bedroom house in Englewood, Colorado. With the family settled, I turned my attention to the Denver Broncos football team, which was not going to leave Denver.

In 1966 when the American Football League merged with the National Football League, no AFL team had ever beaten an NFL team.

The excitement was high in the Mile High City that summer. We beat the Detroit Lions and the Minnesota Vikings on successive weekends in Denver. There were high hopes for the Broncos.

I began learning more about a new kind of hope in Denver. I attended my first Fellowship of Christian Athletes camp in Estes Park, Colorado. I witnessed publicly there for the first time about how Jesus Christ had come into my life. My story, of course, was based on the tragic death of our daughter, Nancy, and how it brought me to Christ. We had also found a Lutheran church in Englewood, and I was teaching during the opening of Sunday school each week. I was no longer a closet Christian. I was, for the first time, able to share my faith. I was tentative but determined. Denver afforded a series of firsts for me.

The first league game was to be against the Boston Patriots, who are now known as the New England Patriots. We jumped out to a 7–0 lead and were on the Patriots' 10-yard line, with less than a yard to go for a touchdown. It was fourth down. I was up in the press box with the headphones on. It was a tense, expectant moment. The crowd was roaring for a touchdown. Lou yelled up to me, asking if we should kick the field goal or go for it. Before I could answer, he screamed, "Let's go for it." He slapped a player on the behind to carry in the play. He didn't wait for my answer. I watched as they came out of the huddle and lined up. With a 7–0 lead, kicking the field goal and taking the safe 3 points should have been the call. I held my breath. The ball was snapped, the lines surged. A brick wall. They stopped us cold.

Lou screamed at me over the headphones, "——, Paul Brown told me never to gamble but to take the points with a field goal. By——, Sam, you're fired!"

"What?!" I was flabbergasted. I couldn't believe it. My first league game in pro football and already I was fired? I never even had a chance to answer Lou's question. I couldn't believe what he was saying to me over the headphones. I didn't even call the play; *he* did. How could I have known then that a similar scene awaited me many years later when I would be the head coach of the Cleveland Browns?

At halftime Lou continued his tirade. *I've heard of emotional coaches, but this is ridiculous,* I thought. I didn't know whether to laugh or cry. If I'd had some money in the bank, I might have seen the humor of the situation.

We were still down 2 points late in the fourth quarter, and I was already rehearsing my speech to Barb. "Hey, Barb, guess what this time? I've been fired during my very first pro league game. Go find us another house somewhere, will you?" I still couldn't believe Lou would say what he did to me. He was still yelling through the headphones, "All we need is 3 points! Get the ball and get a field goal, Sam!" Lou was obviously remembering Paul Brown's advice this time.

As the Patriots bore down on us with a 2-point lead while time was running out, fortune smiled on us. We intercepted a Babe Parilli pass and ran it in for a game-winning touchdown. Great. We won the game, but I was fired. I had all kinds of anxieties while going to the locker room at the end of the game. I showered and dressed immediately because I wanted to get away as soon as possible. I told myself that professional coaching was a rotten business. *Who needs this kind of life anyway? Maybe I ought to go back to college coaching and————*

Lou Saban interrupted my thoughts and put his arms around me, "Sam, I love you!"

"Say what? I thought I was fired."

Lou laughed, "Hey, don't pay any attention to that. That's just the way I am during a game. Half the time I don't even know what I'm saying. We won, didn't we? That's all that counts."

I wondered what would have happened to me if we had lost. It was a great experience for me, however, as I began to understand the monstrous pressures endured by a professional football head coach. I felt a very real compassion for Lou, and I was determined to help him as much as I could. We struggled the rest of the year and lost nine straight games. But we were rebuilding a team, and fortunately, Lou was also the general manager and had a ten-year contract. I also learned that contracts were made to be broken and that there was no such thing as building for the future. Vince Lombardi was right when he said, "Winning isn't everything; it's the only thing." George Allen was also right when he said, "The future is now."

The last game on the Denver schedule was against the Cleveland Browns. A shadow of my future came to me as soon as our 1967 schedule was published. That shadow would lead to real substance in just a few years. It all started when my friend Burt Gottesfeld, a Denver businessman originally from Brooklyn, called me. After saying hello, he said, "Sam, I notice that the Cleveland Browns are scheduled to play Denver in December. You know, Art and Pat Modell are friends of mine, and I'd like you to meet them. How about you and Barb joining us for dinner when they get here?"

I said, "Thanks, that's very nice of you. We'll be happy to meet them."

On Saturday night, prior to the game, Barb and I went to dinner with Art and Pat Modell and Burt. Cleveland won the game. Later I would recall that dinner in Denver when I was interviewed by Art Modell in December 1977.

In the spring of 1968 we found a piece of property on a lake in Littleton, Colorado, in Bow Mar South, a very desirable area. Barb was finally going to have her dream house. Everything looked more permanent to us than it had for years. Lou had a long-term contract, and since it was Lou who had brought me in, I told Barb we could go ahead with the house. She handled the whole thing. With all the experience she's had, she could make it as a general contractor! Of course, she could then sell the houses she built because she has bought and sold so many other ones. She did a terrific job on our new house, but I couldn't help her much because coaching professional football is a seven-day-a-week, twelve-hour-a-day job. Anybody who says otherwise is either naive or lying. I would later find out in 1971 that while moving was difficult, leaving a dream house made it even more difficult.

At Denver we had four so-so years ending in 1970 with no winning seasons. In 1971 John Mazur, head coach of the Boston Patriots, called Lou Saban and asked for permission to negotiate with me. He needed an offensive coordinator. He painted a bright picture because the Patriots were going to draft Jim Plunkett of Stanford University. I flew to Boston at the end of January 1971. John met me at the plane.

"Welcome to Boston, Sam. We'll go right to my office."

In the car we talked about the Broncos for a while, and then John said, "Sam, we're gonna draft Jim Plunkett. I'm sure you know how excited we must be about this."

"Fantastic kid. Won the Heisman. Deserved it, too."

"We've got big plans for him with our team. We're gonna build our whole offense around his passing skills. Terrific arm. He can throw the ball for miles! We want you to help develop him."

"It's exciting just to think about, John. I'd love working with a Heisman Trophy winner. Besides, it's a chance to come back to the East Coast where my family is." The dark side of my thoughts centered on having to tell Barb that we would be moving again and that she would have to give up her dream home in Denver. Saying that she would be upset would be an understatement. *The Music Man*'s Professor Harold Hill would have to sweet-talk her again. I could hear her then, giving me all the reasons we shouldn't move. I had to admit our children were beginning to put down roots at school. The same old tremors started shaking in my stomach.

I returned to Colorado, met with Lou Saban, and talked to some people whose opinions I respected. Everybody—everybody, that is, except Barb—advised me to take the job. Everybody—everybody, that is, except Barb—said I couldn't afford to pass up the opportunity. After four years in her dream house, she had grown to love it and Colorado as well. I knew we would leave a trail of claw marks when we finally left Colorado. Those marks would be made by Barb's fingernails as I dragged her, kicking and screaming, out of her dream house and across the prairie to Boston. After a painful deliberation, without Barb's endorsement, I called and accepted the job from John Mazur. I left on February 1, 1971, and made it back home to Denver only once between February and June. I lived alone in the Sonesta Hotel in Braintree, Massachusetts, for five months. *So this is the fast lane, the big time,* I thought.

# CHAPTER THIRTEEN

# THE FEAR IN THEIR EYES

**B**arb visited Boston in June to search for a house. We had found a town, Holliston, Massachusetts, that suited our needs. The high school had an excellent program and a fine football coach, an important consideration because of Paul's interest in football. He played wide receiver. Jerry Janiskio, a young minister from Elyria, Ohio, was the pastor of a Lutheran church there. Jerry was instrumental in Paul's life. Jerry and I played on the church softball team, and I got involved in his church on a spiritual basis as well. It was the first time I had been so involved in a local church.

Because of our dream house in Denver, Barb wasn't satisfied with any house she saw. We looked at dozens of houses in Holliston and were totally frustrated by the end of the weekend. We finally decided to rent a house. All Barb talked about was the dream house in Denver she had to leave. When that house was sold the first day, we immediately thought it was underpriced. It didn't occur to us at the time that God might be involved in all those dealings. The whole family said good-bye to Denver in the summer of 1971 and moved into our rented house in Holliston.

Our first year at Boston was a great one. Jim Plunkett lived up to his press clippings by breaking many records and being elected Rookie of the Year. Lou Saban had left Denver by this time and had accepted the head coaching job at Buffalo. I had a number of opportunities that year but decided to stay with the Patriots. However, we did manage to move again—from the rented house to one we bought. Barb, once again, had to do all the moving.

In 1972 we had high hopes. High hopes, that is, until October when the Patriots played the Dolphins in Miami. The Dolphins had an abundance of talent on that team. Don Shula was their coach, and it was the beginning of the Shula dynasty. Larry Csonka, Paul Warfield, and Bob Griese were on a roll. I was in the press box while John Mazur paced the sidelines. They scored immediately and then rolled up a 51–0 score. They tore us apart, and that's putting it mildly.

After the game, something strange happened. As I walked off the field, I heard a noise coming from the stands, growing in volume and building like the roar of a hundred airplanes approaching. I turned around and looked up into the stands. Thousands of people were chanting Don Shula's name. "Shu-la! Shu-la! Shu-la!" I shook my head and walked the rest of the way to the locker room.

I'll never forget that sight or those sounds. I knew that John Mazur was going to be fired. It was an eerie and foreboding knowledge because I began to sense more of the uncertainties of the coaching profession. The next day John Mazur called a meeting of all the coaches and dramatically announced that he had been fired. I looked around at all the other assistant coaches and saw the fear in their eyes. Our collective futures were in doubt. What would we all do about our families? the schools for our children? My first thought was that Paul was going to be a senior in high school. If we had to move once again, he would have to attend a new high school in his senior year. It would be a great disappointment to him. How could I ask him to move now? His team had been state champions two years in a row. He had been looking forward to his senior year as any young man would.

It suddenly hit me that this was the way it was in professional football. Mazur's dismissal was a great test. Some coaches and many players wanted to fold their tents and quit—and you found out whether or not you really wanted to coach. It was my first experience as a lame-duck coach who faced the strong possibility of being let go at the end of the season.

Phil Bengtson, former head coach for the Green Bay Packers, came in as interim head coach for the final five games of the 1972 season. The rest of us were retained for the balance of the season with the probability that we would be fired when it was over. I watched as each assistant coach tried to deal with the dilemma in his own way. I learned that if you really wanted to coach at this level, you had to make the total commitment—even if you were going to be dismissed at the end of five weeks. I decided that I would give it the best I could and not worry beyond that. We had a season to finish. As it turned out, we won only one more game out of the five. It was simply a miserable season.

All the coaches were in a holding pattern while we waited for owner

Billy Sullivan to name a new coach. Names like Joe Paterno of Penn State and Bob Devaney of Nebraska were rumored. At the end of January, three days before the player draft, Chuck Fairbanks, head coach of the University of Oklahoma, was hired. The press conference was on a Friday, and that Friday night he met with John Mazur's staff. He went around the room asking each assistant coach to talk about each player he had coached.

When I left that meeting and started driving home, I felt empty and hopeless about my future in professional football. I arrived home and explained everything to Barb and the kids. It seemed certain that I would be fired. The hazards of coaching filled my mind. I thought about Harry Ostro, the former coach at Lafayette High School, who gave me my first head coaching job. He said, "The difference between a pat on the back and a kick in the tail is six inches. When you win, you get a pat; when you lose, you get the kick."

The next day, all the assistant coaches were in their respective offices. We knew Chuck Fairbanks was going to call each of us into his office and give a token interview before he fired us. I sat there feeling like a man on death row on the day he was scheduled to die. One by one, Chuck called the coaches into his office. One by one, each coach left Chuck's office and walked silently by my door straight back to his own office and began to pack his personal belongings. Finally it was my turn. When Chuck called me, my gut did a somersault. Those few steps to his office were my personal "last mile." Because I knew him slightly, I found it difficult to talk to Chuck. He was a quiet man and very hard for me to read. I swallowed hard and walked into his office. I was determined to sell him on his need for my services.

"Congratulations, Chuck. No matter what happens, I want to wish you luck. I realize that you must have a number of prospective coaches in mind."

He surprised me with his opening statement, "I'd like you to stay, Sam. You can help me as a football coach, but just as important, I want someone who has values such as you have on my staff."

Relief flooded into my chest. It was an emotional mixed bag. I was elated that we wouldn't have to move, that Paul would be able to finish out his senior year at his high school. I wouldn't have to tell Barb to call United Van Lines again! But I would have to face the rest of the coaching staff who were my buddies. *Why was I the only one retained on the staff?* I asked myself. I didn't view myself as any better than the rest of the guys. They were all proficient at their jobs. My curiosity began to grow about this strange good luck of mine. I found out why when the owner, Billy Sullivan, walked up to me that same day and said, "Congratulations, Sam. We're all pleased that you're going to stay with us. You may be interested to know that Peter Hadhazy gave you a strong endorsement. He told us that you had a lot to do with Plunkett's development and that Plunkett wanted you to stay." So that was why they kept me on. Peter Hadhazy was the assistant general manager who was retained as Chuck Fairbanks's right-hand man. He and I were good friends. This relationship would be important to me some years later when the Cleveland Browns came knocking on my door.

Even during all the changes, I was reminded once again how tenuous the life of a coach can be. Not more than a few weeks later, I was approached by the Montreal Alouettes, of the Canadian Football League, to be their head coach. When the owner of the Alouettes called me, I knew he had already received permission from Chuck Fairbanks to talk with me. I really wasn't interested, but the offer gave me something to think about. After thinking it through, I realized there were two important reasons I wasn't interested: first, I didn't want to move because of Paul's senior year, and second, I didn't want to get out of the mainstream of the NFL. My decision not to accept the offer was the first I had made that was influenced more by family needs than by personal ambition. As it turned out, my staying was difficult because it placed me in the middle of a lot of talk about all the mistakes the previous coaching staff had made. I felt a loyalty to my former coaching peers, and yet I knew I should be totally loyal to Chuck. I didn't mention it to Barb, but I already knew I would leave the Patriots at the end of the season. It was just another loser.

# CHAPTER FOURTEEN

# CALLING ME HOME

**A**s a high-school coach, I had often fantasized about coaching in New York City on the professional level. In 1974 Bill Arnsparger was head coach of the Giants, and Charley Winner was head coach of the Jets.

I knew Charley Winner from having attended a Fellowship for Christian Athletes camp with him in Estes Park, Colorado, in the late sixties when he was head coach for the St. Louis Cardinals. In 1974, both Charley and Bill were offering to hire me. I opted for the Jets. Their offer was intriguing because it was a chance to coach the defensive secondary. That would give me the experience on the other side of the ball that was so essential in preparing myself to be a head coach.

But telling my sweet wife was a monumental problem. I went home and bit the bullet. "Barb, I've just been offered a coaching job with the Jets."

"Sam, you can't do that. You've got a job with the Patriots."

"Not any more. We're going to New York."

"Sam, you can't be serious. We've been here only two years! I just finished decorating this house. We can't go anywhere."

"Now, Barb——"

"Now, Barb?! Now, Barb?! I've heard *that* before. The kids are settled in school, the house is terrific, you get home once in awhile. If you go to New York, we won't see you for six months except on weekends. I don't know why a woman wants to be a coach's wife anyway. Oh, Sam, I love this house. I don't want to leave it."

Every Monday morning at four o'clock I traveled from Boston to New York. Every Friday afternoon I traveled from New York to Boston. Since the Jets didn't provide for any housing, I slept on a cot in the locker room at Shea Stadium. Because my mother lived nearby in Brooklyn, I was able to have dinner with her once each week. Even if I had been fired by a football team or two, at least Mom was always happy to have me around!

The first night, I tossed around on the cot for a long time. Cots were for kids, I decided. I finally went to sleep, but not for long. I awakened with a start and knew something was wrong. I looked all around in the dark but could see nothing. I knew I had heard something. It was loud enough to awaken me. Maybe thieves were in the stadium. It was like being in a dark cave. Then suddenly there was a loud noise. My hair stood up. That wasn't my imagination! That was real. Something was going on.

I didn't want to leave the locker room because I didn't know my way around the place. I didn't know if anyone else was allowed in there at night, but I was sure someone else was inside the stadium. I felt helpless and defenseless. I looked around for some kind of weapon. When I found a Louisville Slugger, I felt a bit better. A long period of time went by, and the noises stopped. I lay down again with the bat beside me. I was almost asleep again when *blam!* Something seemed to crash against something else in the stadium. I jumped up again and grabbed the bat while my heart pumped up. I listened, poised with bat in hand, ready to swing. Nothing. I took a deep breath and lay down again, nervous as a cornered rat, and finally went to sleep. I made it through the night not knowing what caused the noises. The security people told me the next day that the noises were caused by people trying to break in. I slept with one eye open and the Louisville Slugger on my cot for the rest of the spring. When Barb came to New York so that we could search for a house, we certainly didn't stay in the stadium. I made other arrangements for her visits.

Mrs. Pallmeyer was still living in Huntington where Barb had lived for two and a half years. That was one good point helping to sway Barb to move. She would be able to visit her often. They loved each other very much. So Barb was elated to find a house in Huntington Bay close to Mrs. Pallmeyer. We made an offer on the house just three hours before we had to return to Boston. Just as we were leaving Mrs. Pallmeyer, the phone rang. The realtor said that the owners had accepted our offer. That move was the most pleasant in our career because we were returning to home territory. After all the difficult moves, we finally engineered one that Barb liked. If she liked it, I liked it.

In the interim between January and June, Barb sold the Holliston house for a profit. She was slowly but surely becoming expert in the buying and selling of real estate. She was looking forward to renewing her close friendship with Mrs. Pallmeyer when we moved to Huntington at the end of June. But the dust had no more than settled when we received some very bad news. Mrs. Pallmeyer had suffered a severe stroke. We had been in our new house only a week when her son moved her to a hospital care center in Saint Louis. It was a sad day for all of us. Barb would have been very glad to help care for her had Mrs. Pallmeyer stayed in her home close by. With our dear friend gone, we turned our attention to finding a church where we could find some new friends. We found just that at Saint Peter's Lutheran Church, the same church where Barb and I were married.

When I first reported for work with the Jets at Shea Stadium, I was as excited as any fan would be to meet and work with Joe Namath. He was already a big star in football, television, radio, and movies. But I discovered a side of Broadway Joe that was never made public. Once he reported to training camp and started concentrating exclusively on football, he was one of the most dedicated and hard-working players I had ever worked with. He was also one of the toughest, most competitive, intelligent players I ever knew. He was very friendly, personable and, believe it or not, shy. He would stand patiently for hours after practice signing autographs. Privately he helped many teammates and former teammates and friends financially.

When Charley Winner was finally fired, Joe Namath said to me, "Charley is the first coach who ever got fired during the time I played for him." Joe always shouldered the blame when things got tough, no matter if it involved a player or a coach. He always took full responsibility and never said anything negative about anyone.

There was a mystique about Joe Namath and the way the other players responded to his leadership. It was so obvious when he was on the field that our guys tried their very best while Joe called the plays. He expected the best from each player, and they wanted to give it for him. I first realized this when the backup quarterback, Al Woodall, went in when Joe was hurt. Al was a very fine quarterback who could have played on any NFL team, but Al would be the first to tell you that Joe's ability to inspire men to extraordinary action was there for everyone to see. When Joe first started to emerge as a nationally known personality, many people thought he was all showboat.

The first time I saw Joe getting suited up for a game was a revelation to me. His knee braces extended from the middle of his calves to the middle of his thighs. He played with pain almost all the time. Yet he could take the snap from center and fade back to the pocket as fast as anyone else in the league. I was absolutely amazed at how all players and coaches, including our opponents, respected Joe's ability. Even my sweet wife was mesmerized by Joe's charm.

During my first Jet training camp at Hofstra University in Hempstead, New York, Barb stopped by to pick me up after our coaches' meeting. Just as she walked up the sidewalk, Joe came out of the dorm. I introduced them, and I stood there watching my dear wife react like I had just introduced her to Clark Gable. She started talking and never stopped. Joe had that effect on women.

When the New York Jets football campaign started in 1974, we lost seven of the first eight games we played. The rumors were already starting. But we played our next game against the New York Giants, and we beat them in overtime. We won the next six games. I particularly enjoyed our win over my former team, the Patriots, that year because we intercepted Plunkett four times and I was awarded the game ball. We finished the season on a strong note, and our prospects were bright for 1975. Joe Namath had a great year and was talking about 1975 the way he had talked about the 1969 Super Bowl when he predicted the Jets would win it all.

We went into the 1975 training camp with high hopes. Those hopes turned into despair when the players decided to strike. Everything was suddenly on hold. We missed the entire preseason with our veteran players. The NFL owners decided to play the preseason with rookies and free agents, regardless of where they came from. We were so desperate for players that we actually held tryouts.

One night Charley Winner and his wife, Nancy, ran into a kid who was working behind the counter in a pizza place. When Charley learned that he had some experience as a receiver, he recruited him on the spot. The kid threw off his apron and took off with Charley. He switched from slinging pizzas to catching footballs. He was on the roster that weekend when we journeyed to Denver and beat them in a preseason game. It was a trying time but a very rewarding experience coaching kids literally off the streets. The problem was that they began to fantasize about being permanent professional football players.

To get players for those preseason games we were willing to try almost anything. Once a young man showed up on the practice field in Hempstead, New York, in a business suit. He wanted so badly to try out that he began stripping right there. I watched incredulously as he opened his briefcase, took out a pair of running shoes, and promptly ran the 40-yard dash for us. The kid was fast. We signed him before he could get away.

Some of the young men who showed up were long on confidence but short on talent. The worst performance I witnessed during those "tryouts" was by a young man who was so slow, he couldn't run 40 yards in thirty minutes. He didn't run, he waddled. Johnny Carson might ask, "How slow was he?" He was so slow it would take him two green lights to cross the street. I tried to break the news to him gently, but he couldn't handle the rejection. He became enraged and promptly urinated on all the newly planted bushes around the field. Almost anybody else would have yelled or swung at me or at least foamed at the mouth, but his reaction was a first. We quickly stopped the tryouts because we didn't know what the nut might do next. I've always said urination was better than assassination. I still haven't figured out why he chose the bushes. Those were trying times, indeed.

The player strike was finally settled, but something was very wrong with our team. Many of the guys were heavily involved in the union struggle, and they simply weren't ready to start the season. Most of the other teams were way ahead of us in conditioning and attitudes. Many of our players were bitter. It's tough enough to succeed in the NFL when all the guys are pulling together. Most of them didn't even want to work out. Joe Namath got so upset about it that he left town. He just couldn't handle it. He was sympathetic with the players, but he couldn't understand why they didn't want to work out and keep in shape, strike or no strike. He recognized that they would be investing in their own future by keeping in shape. Everybody, especially a star like Joe Namath, knew that conditioning was as important as God-given talent. I've always had great respect for Joe because he played on those painful, wobbly knees of his. So the team and the season went right down the drain. With just a few games to go, Charley Winner was fired. The owners elevated Ken Shipp from offensive coordinater to interim head coach. There I was again, three years later, a lame-duck coach.

Shortly after that, we invited one of the coaches, Mike Holovak, who was separated, to dinner at our home. Barb, like most females, was always sensitive about the appearance of her home. While we were in the middle of eating dinner, Barb said something that would cause most males to chuckle.

Barb smiled and said, "Mike, I hope you'll forgive me for not having curtains hung in the living room."

Poor Mike was caught off guard, "Huh? Oh, ah, hey, Barb, I hadn't even noticed. I mean——"

"I'm going to have them installed right away, but I've been so busy lately."

"Well, hey, don't do that on my account. Besides, you might as well save your energy because we're all going to get fired anyway."

I watched Barb's face. I could have choked Mike. I hadn't told Barb yet about how bad things were with the Jets. I couldn't believe my ears. My buddy, Mike, was torpedoing me in my own home! Barb stared daggers at me all the rest of the evening. It was a tense time. When Mike left, I had a big job of explaining to do.

Sure enough, two weeks later, all of us got fired. The season ended on a dismal note because we didn't win a single game after Charley Winner was fired. I felt my career and hopes of becoming a head coach slipping away.

But then Ron Perry, athletic director at Holy Cross, called me and asked if I would be interested in interviewing for the head coaching job at Holy Cross. It would mean moving back to Boston. Although it wasn't the NFL, it was a head coaching position. I had begun to see that the only way to have any control over my destiny in this crazy business was to become a head coach on *any* level. The interview process went extremely well, and it looked as if the job was mine if I wanted it. The last step was a chat with Father Brooks, the president of Holy Cross College, a very nice man. I asked him how important football would be in a small, private Catholic college. He answered, "The students need something they can identify with in the fall of the year."

I immediately knew that Father Brooks and I were not on the same page. I proceeded to voice my views, and with each comment the job went further down the drain. I left the informal "chat" knowing full well that there would be no move back to Boston.

Although I had a year left on my contract with the Jets, I told them I wouldn't return, no matter who they got as a head coach. Lo and behold, Lou Holtz was hired away from North Carolina State to take over the job for the Jets. Beth Holtz called Barb and wanted to visit us and see our house, which was for sale. It seemed we *always* had a house for sale. Barb made coffee and cake, and they are still waiting. The Holtzes never showed up. It was just as well because I never would sell my house to a coach. I would be too sympathetic with the poor slob and probably give the house away. Everybody knows what the game of musical chairs is. Coaches play musical houses throughout their entire careers.

All our other moves were only preludes to what turned out to be Barb's most difficult move. I had been in the NFL nine years and had moved four times, and another move was imminent. But this was to be my "last move." If this situation didn't work out, I was going to return to New York and find other employment. I would take my father's advice and "get a real job."

I was hired by the New Orleans Saints, but I wasn't totally enthusiastic about the job. I was getting a bellyfull of being an assistant coach and moving around the country like a yo-yo. Poor Barb was so touchy about all the hirings and firings that she decided it would be best not to sell our house in New York. "That way," she said, "we'll have a house to return to when you get fired by the Saints." She didn't say "if" you get fired, she said "when." What other profession offers you almost a guarantee of being fired the very day you're hired? We reported to New Orleans with our tails dragging but looking hopefully toward that dim light at the end of the tunnel. After all those years, I had almost forgotten that light always follows darkness.

# CHAPTER FIFTEEN

# I WILL GET READY, MY CHANCE WILL COME

Joining the New Orleans Saints proved to be the turning point of my coaching career. Even before reporting to New Orleans in January 1976, I had decided to get out of football altogether if the job didn't work out. Although I was a believer in Christ, I wasn't obedient. I didn't know how to be obedient. But, somehow, I began to suspect that God had more to do with my moves than I realized.

We bought our eighth house in Covington, Louisiana, which was located on the other side of a twenty-four-mile causeway across Lake Pontchartrain. When the realtor told the seller that I was a coach with the New Orleans Saints, he said, "He'll need that twenty-four miles of water to separate himself from the fans because the Saints are going to lose a lot of games."

New Orleans was the only NFL team that never had been in the playoffs or had a winning season. I had high hopes because Hank Stram had accepted the head coaching job, and it appeared that he knew how to turn the team into a winner. Archie Manning, the quarterback, was the key factor. But our season never got off the ground because Manning injured his arm and missed the entire season. What a blow! Our train never got out of the station.

Close to the end of the season, I was seriously thinking of quitting football for good. The pain was just too prolonged and fulfillment too elusive. Of course, I didn't know then that the lasting fulfillment for which I was searching couldn't be found simply by winning football games. I was about to give up when I received a telephone call from John Toner, the athletic director at the University of Connecticut. During the Christmas holidays, I flew to Storrs, Connecticut, and was interviewed for the job. It looked good to me even though it would never lead to the Rose Bowl or big-time football. As I walked around the campus, I sensed the old attraction of the college scene that had never quite left me. Deep down I still viewed myself as a college football coach. It was like a call to return home to my old stamping ground. When I left the campus that day, I was sure the job was mine if I wanted it.

I flew back to New Orleans determined to make this a family decision. I told Barb, "The NFL is just not for me. This college offer seems just right. I'm sure it'll be best for the family. We'll make it our *final* move. We'll buy a house in Storrs, and I'll spend the rest of my working days at the college level of coaching."

I wasn't prepared for Barb's answer, "Sam, who are you trying to kid? Why would you want to quit after all these moves and steps toward accomplishing your life's goal? Six months into the job in Connecticut and you'll be miserable. I know you. The opportunity passed for Connecticut years ago. Why not keep on trying in the pros? Someday you'll make it, Sam. You'll reach your goal and become a head coach in the NFL."

Was this my Barb? Was this the same Barb I'd always heard moan about all the moves? I said, "I thought you'd be happy to hear I'd given up on the NFL. I thought you'd like it if I went back to the college scene."

"Sam, why quit when you might be close? Look at all the experience you've had. Some owner will need you one of these days. There aren't too many coaches around with your experience."

Barb's words seemed to be exactly what I needed to hear. It was almost like the after-shave commercial. I felt like saying, "Thanks, I needed that." After thinking about the Connecticut offer a little longer, I called to turn it down. I put the idea of quitting my coaching career on a back burner. Still I couldn't put it entirely out of my mind. I would wait a little longer and see what might happen.

By the middle of the 1977 season, we were trying our best to lose most of our games. Already I was sorry I passed up the University of Connecticut offer. With two games left, rumors were flying around New Orleans that Hank Stram's days were numbered. Our thirteenth game was to be against the Tampa Bay Buccaneers who had lost twenty-eight straight games. We were sure to win it, right? Wrong! We were running scared during our week-long preparation for that game. I was almost totally depressed that week about the upcoming game, about coaching, about life itself. There I was, certain to be fired, along with Hank, once again. I went home on Thursday night worn out and full of self-pity. Barb met me at the door.

"Sam, Peter Hadhazy called. He wants you to call him back."

"I wonder what Pete wants. He probably wants to buck me up. Or maybe he wants to place a bet or something. Of all the games we're supposed to win, it's this one against Tampa Bay." I was depressed enough at that moment to appreciate a call from an old friend. Pete and I had become close during our days with the Patriots. He was now the executive vice president and general manager of the Cleveland Browns. I dialed his number. Pete came right to the point.

"Sam, they're going to ask Forrest Gregg to resign before the last game of the season. How would you like to be the head coach for the Cleveland Browns? I feel very strongly that Art Modell will listen to my recommendation and bring you to Cleveland for an interview after our final game. Are you interested?"

I could hardly believe what I was hearing. My tongue seemed to be twisted around my teeth. I was like a man who had fallen overboard from a ship and was being offered a life raft. Was I interested? "Sure, Pete. Sure I'm interested."

"Sam, it's very important that everything be kept in the strictest confidence. Sam, I'm telling you that the job is yours if you don't blow the interview!"

I thanked Pete, put the telephone down, and stood there stunned. Had I really heard right? Was I dreaming? Just when I was at my lowest ebb in life, the sun broke through. Hope, sweet hope, flooded through my soul. I rushed to the kitchen.

"Barb, how would you like to be the First Lady?"

"What are you talking about?"

"You aren't going to believe this. Pete Hadhazy just called and said Art Modell wants to interview me for the head coaching job for the Cleveland Browns. Can you believe it?"

"Sam, I told you all along that God would take care of us. I'm not surprised at all."

I stared at my wife. She was only five feet two inches tall, but at that moment she seemed to be as tall and strong as the Statue of Liberty. It seemed that the longer we lived together, the more I appreciated her. But then a sudden fear gripped me. I said, "Oh, my gosh, what if we lose to Tampa Bay this Sunday? How could Peter sell me to the Cleveland media if we lose to them? After all, assistant coaches who take over head coaching jobs usually come from Super Bowl teams." I was really worried. Besides that, I began to feel guilty about being the only one on the Saints staff with a ticket on the lifeboat out of New Orleans.

As I waited for the game day to arrive, my worries had grown to huge proportions because I had a feeling we were going to lose. Modell would probably watch at least part of our game and tell Pete to forget me. I felt like I was dying.

The big day came on Sunday when we lined up against Tampa Bay. I kept remembering that they had lost twenty-eight straight games. *How could we lose to them?* I asked myself. I didn't have to wait long for an answer. By the time the first quarter was over, I knew the dike had broken and water was flooding the city. They clobbered us. I couldn't believe the score: Tampa Bay 33, New Orleans 14. I couldn't believe that Cleveland could still be interested in me after the unbelievable loss to Tampa Bay. That night I was afraid to go to any restaurant because the fans might murder me. I was afraid to go home because I didn't want to hear Peter Hadhazy explain over the telephone why Cleveland really didn't want to talk to me after all. I could picture Pete pleading my case to Modell who was probably shaking his head at that moment. So, I took Barb and the girls to McDonald's.

Finally we went home, but no call came. I went to work Monday and still no call. At home that night, I was getting ready to watch "Monday Night Football" on television when the phone rang. It was Peter Hadhazy.

"Sam, we're really anxious to get you up here for an interview. Art Modell is going to call John Mecom for permission to talk with you. They're considering Joe Paterno, Ara Parseghian, and Joe Restic, but you're the guy who is going to get the job."

I put the phone down and still couldn't believe what I had just heard. After all the years of preparation, with some thrills of victory and many agonizing defeats, of learning and relearning, days of joy and nights of despair, suddenly my goal was within reach. Already I was thinking like a head coach and considering which of my fellow coaches I would invite to Cleveland with me. It was as if I knew exactly what to do and how to proceed. I had waited so long for this to happen. I knew how it would feel to those I picked and to those I left behind. My mind was spinning into high gear. But our season in New Orleans wasn't quite over.

Our final game was in Atlanta. On Saturday night, before the game on Sunday, I had a fever of 103 degrees. I worked through the game (which we lost), but I was determined to go to Cleveland on Monday, no matter what my health condition was.

Late Monday morning, Hank Stram called me into his office and said, "Sam, the Cleveland Browns have asked permission to interview you. It looks like a great opportunity for you. I've been through several interviews like that. I know Art Modell, and I believe he's a good man. You might say the Cleveland Browns organization is the flagship of the fleet when you consider their past record."

As Hank and I talked, I appreciated his graciousness. I went back to my office and called Pete. He said, "Sam, get a flight to Cleveland on Tuesday afternoon. When you land, get your bags and look outside for Art Modell's Mercedes sedan with a chauffeur named Joe Harris. He'll pick you up and drive you to the Sheraton Hotel located at Route 306 and I-90 in Mentor, Ohio. You'll register under an alias. Relax until Joe picks you up to join Art and Pat Modell and Rita and me for dinner at Art's home in Waite Hill, Ohio. It's very close to the hotel."

Alias! Wasn't that illegal or something? I had never used an alias before in my entire life. At the hotel desk I felt like 007. I looked around to see if any reporters were lurking in the lobby. It was exciting. I couldn't wait to arrive at Art's house. I had never looked forward to anything so much as the upcoming meeting.

In my room I was ready very soon and found myself pacing the floor, looking out the window, and pacing the floor some more. I prayed a lot, too. I called Barb and told her to keep praying. She said she had been praying all day. Not long afterward I found myself being driven to Art's home in his Mercedes. It seemed as if only five minutes passed before we arrived.

The dinner was nice and informal. We were getting to know each other. Meanwhile my mind was racing as I tried to anticipate the questions Art might ask. We talked a lot about football, of course, but nothing about my proposed offer. The suspense was high for me.

After dinner we sat in the Modell's living room and enjoyed a warm conversation. Art was from Brooklyn, so we had much in common. Pat was from New York City, also. It was almost like old home week. The atmosphere was congenial, and as the evening continued, Art became more and more transparent. He shared his great disappointment about the way the team was going. I could tell then that he really wanted his new coach to be someone who would understand his position as an owner, someone who could become his friend. He seemed to have a poignant longing to have a family relationship with his team. He often referred to the players as his kids. I was touched by his sincerity. I was aware of being in the presence of a quality human being. I didn't realize it then, but I came to understand that what Art sincerely wanted was an impossibility in the world of professional sports.

He talked that night about players and coaches who, in "the old days," would give their word and their right hand as pledges to a contract. He lamented what he considered to be a legalistic approach with agents, highly paid players, and all the rest. It was almost as if he was thinking of throwing it all over. I deeply appreciated his openness because I was able to share some of my own deep feelings. Both of us had been experiencing periods of disappointment, and I felt a close bond beginning to form between us. We seemed to view each other as a source of new hope. It was a good evening and one filled with high hopes for me. Pete Hadhazy really went to bat for me. Art wanted me to return to his home the next day. As I rode back to the hotel, I felt better than I had felt in years. *This is what I've been waiting for all my life. I just know it.*

Back in the hotel that night I called Barb and told her that I believed the interview was the best I ever had. I was too excited to fall asleep right away.

The next morning I returned to Art's house for breakfast and stayed all day. Art, Peter Hadhazy, and I spent the entire day talking, discussing offense and defense, watching films, and trying to plan ahead. By the end of the day, I really felt confident that Art was going to make me an offer. He said he had planned to talk to some other candidates, but I had the feeling that he had already made up his mind. Also, during that day, I got the distinct impression that, if I was hired, Art wanted to build a solid friendship as well. I was elated because it's my nature to develop friendships with almost anyone who wants to do so. I've always been an outgoing person. It was a real plus to me because Art wanted to be a friend to his head coach. Neither of us could have known then the anguish our friendship would cause us later.

Peter took me to the airport, and I flew home to await the phone call. Don't ask me how the word had gotten out so soon that I was being considered for the Cleveland job. I had no idea there were so many people interested in whether or not I was going to become the next head coach for the Cleveland Browns. I wanted the line to stay clear for Pete's call, but all day long the phone rang. I received a lot of free advice that day. If I had listened to everyone who had recommended assistant coaches for me to hire, we might have needed the Los Angeles Memorial Coliseum for the first staff meeting.

I waited a couple of days, which seemed to be an eternity. On Christmas Eve I was sitting in the family room talking to the family when the telephone rang. I can still hear Art Modell's words in my memory. I still appreciate the classy way in which he gave me the good news. When I answered the telephone, Art said, "May I speak to the head coach of the Cleveland Browns, please?"

*Merry Christmas, Rutiglianos,* I thought. How appropriate to receive such a call on Christmas Eve. I breathed a prayer of thanks knowing where and from whom the new opportunity had really come.

# CHAPTER SIXTEEN

# SAM WHO?

When I was appointed head coach of the Cleveland Browns, I didn't realize how difficult it would be to put a staff together. I also never realized that I knew so many people in coaching. I got calls from all over the United States. The phones never stopped ringing in my New Orleans home and at the Browns' office. I couldn't keep up with all the messages. I decided, however, to organize and answer all of them one way or the other. I vowed that I would treat people as best I could on the way "up" because I might meet them again on the way down. I knew how it felt to be on both ends of the ladder.

I learned a lot during that time in my life. I learned that the quest for popularity ends once you assume the responsibility of directing others. What a problem. There were only eight to ten positions available on my staff, and I had many friends who wanted to join the Browns with me. Unfortunately, some relationships were never the same after I made the selections.

I flew back to Cleveland between Christmas and New Year's Eve to attend a press conference at Cleveland Municipal Stadium, the same place I was destined to be when I got fired on October 21, 1984. I stayed at Art Modell's house where he protected me from everybody for a while. Pat Modell was cordial and couldn't have been nicer to me. It was obvious that Pat had a major influence on Art. She was good for him. She had that inner talent to judge people. Sometimes women can actually jump over the facts and make solid judgments. I admired Pat's toughness and intense loyalty to Art.

The press conference went well. Art said it was the best that he had ever attended. He had attended five at that point, and neither he nor I knew that there were going to be more. Art had fired four coaches by the time he hired me. To paraphrase Samuel Johnson when he referred to second marriages: "It is the triumph of hope over experience." But all beginnings are like honeymoons. Sooner or later, all honeymoons end. What a fun job, this coaching. As Bum Phillips once said, "The day you're hired is one day closer to the day you'll be fired. Coaching is not a job in which you grow old gracefully. It's as easy as replacing a light bulb. As soon as one burns out, it's that much easier to plug in another one." After eleven years in the pros, I already knew the truth of Bum's statement. If only you didn't have to win all the time. If you just didn't have to show up on Sundays and play the games, it would be a fun job. I did have a lot of fun at the press conference because I was doing the thing I did best: communicating.

At that press conference many reporters asked me who had negotiated my contract. I told them there would be no problem with my contract because Art had negotiated my contract with my Uncle Vito who had made Art an offer he just couldn't refuse!

They asked a lot of questions, but one I heard the most was "Sam Who?" They didn't really know much about me, even though I had spent eleven years with four different NFL teams: Denver, New England, the New York Jets, and New Orleans. The best record I could put my finger on was in New York in 1974 when we were 7–7. I was "Sam Who." I had spent eleven years in the NFL and had not had a winning season. Head coaches in the NFL were usually chosen from Super Bowl teams, football's Knights of the Round Table. Or you had to be a genius like Bill Arnsparger or Howard Schnellenberger from the Miami Dolphins staff or a Bill Walsh from the Cincinnati staff. Coaches from losing teams just didn't get jobs in the NFL. It was great for me when Peter Hadhazy jumped up on a table and stomped his feet in my behalf. But more than anything, the confidence Art Modell displayed gave me the biggest boost. I came to Cleveland with the idea of really being free. I was aware of these words during that press conference: "The LORD is my helper; I will not fear." What could man do to me if the Lord be for me? The very worst thing that could happen would be my losing my address.

Meantime, Barb was back in New Orleans trying to sell still another house. Then she had to come to Cleveland to find another one. It meant another six months' separation from my family. I counted the months we had been separated in the last eight years. The total came to two whole years! I couldn't believe it. I moved from Denver to Boston during the spring of 1971; from Boston to New York during the spring of

1974; from New York to New Orleans during the spring of 1976; and from New Orleans to Cleveland during the spring of 1978. People talk about quality time. What a lot of baloney! There's no such thing as quality time. There is just time. In life, we can't call any time-outs. All we have left is time.

At draft time, we had two number-one draft choices. We had traded Mike Phipps to the Chicago Bears for their number-one choice. Our first selection was Clay Matthews, who became a Pro Bowl linebacker with the Browns. Our second pick, late in the first round, was Ozzie Newsome. He was a split end on the wishbone, a run-oriented offense, at the University of Alabama. We felt that Ozzie had the build of a tight end, and he was very agreeable to playing that position. He said that the late Bear Bryant had already told him that he would be a great tight end in the NFL.

I watched many dramatic scenes from the sideline as Ozzie broke open and Brian Sipe found him. The 1978 team electrified the crowd. They screamed constantly as, time after time, Brian sailed that football and Ozzie made a leaping, diving catch. It didn't take long for everyone to realize why Ozzie was known as the Wizard of Oz. He had glue fingers. He could leap up and hold onto the ball, stretch out horizontally and hold onto the ball, dive down and hold onto the ball. He could catch a BB in the dark. I always loved running to meet him and yelling, "Nice catch, Ozzie." We developed the tight-end screen because of Ozzie's talent. It was always exciting to watch, and Ozzie did it so well.

I loved meeting all the players as they came off the field after a good play, slapping each one on the behind and saying, "Way to go." As a touchdown play unfolded, I was like a little kid, running along the sideline and watching the ball fly through the air to Ozzie or Reggie Rucker or any of the other receivers in the end zone. I jumped up and down, clapped my hands, yelled praises to our players, feeling the laughter welling up in me and coming out. Man, it was exhilarating! There's no feeling like it.

A coach lives and dies a thousand deaths on the sideline during a game. During the heat and pressure of a game with the crowd screaming all the time, a coach has only a few seconds to make a call. It sounds like double-talk sometimes, but it has to be in "code." When that clock is ticking, you have to spit it out fast like, "Brown right, nasty, slant 135, 94 fullback banana, hot right." Or "Dive 32" or "Double tight end, pick 38" or "Brown right, lag 242." That's why it's so important for the players to know the playbook.

But sometimes it takes more than knowing the playbook. You've got to have a little luck here and there. Ozzie knew the playbook very well. There were times that year when Ozzie made great catches only to have the play called back. Maybe they thought because I was a rookie head coach I wouldn't scream at the refs. Bad calls are part of the game, but they sure give ulcers to coaches. That year, I yelled at the refs plenty. I remember one such robbery when a Sipe-to-Newsome play got called back. I saw a defensive tackle holding one of our players, but the ref didn't see it. I yelled to the ref, "Hey, Ref, he's been holding all day long! He literally tackled the fullback! He tackled him, for cryin' out loud! Open your eyes, Ref! I can't believe this guy!" Now everybody knows there's nothing disrespectful about that! Any self-respecting coach would do it.

Yes, the Sipe-to-Newsome drama started in 1978 when Ozzie was a rookie. He has, since that time, caught more passes than any other NFL tight end. He's already destined for the Pro Football Hall of Fame in Canton, Ohio, which is appropriately located only fifty miles south of Cleveland, new home for the Rutigliano family.

Barb and I fell in love with the East Side of Cleveland. It had Italian restaurants and Jewish delicatessens everywhere. It reminded us of Brooklyn. We engaged Helen Richardson, Art Modell's realtor, who found us a house on eleven acres in Waite Hill, Ohio. Waite Hill, like Chagrin Falls and Hudson, Ohio, is almost more New Englandish than New England itself. We loved the house, which was located very close to Art Modell's house. The unique thing about this home purchase was that I bought it before Barb saw it.

Training camp was exciting, but our season was about to open, which meant that the honeymoon was over. No matter how good my relationship with Art was, it would last only if we won. Our first game was with the San Francisco 49ers at Cleveland Municipal Stadium. A lot of my friends came to the opener. Frank and Joe Torre, two baseball friends from Brooklyn, reminded me how important it was to get off to a good start. Many of the kids from Lafayette High days came to the game to cheer me on. They were true friends.

We beat San Francisco that day. It was a grand day. Brian Sipe and Ozzie Newsome were impressive.

I found out that Brian was the youngest player as a catcher on a Little League team that went to Williamsport, Pennsylvania, and won the Little League World Series. Brian had been supercompetitive since he was a little kid. I loved it. Don Coryell, who coached Brian in college, told me, "He'll battle for you." It was my first game as a head coach in the NFL and Ozzie's first pro game. Brian and Ozzie really clicked that day.

I had spent a lot of time trying to find out as much as possible about Brian Sipe. He was the most competitive football player, regardless of position, I had ever known. He was intelligent, creative, and tough, and he was at his best in crucial situations. We were destined to have many last-minute wins engineered by Brian. When he came to the sideline during those time-outs close to the end of the games, he always gave me that feeling of utmost confidence. The tighter the circumstances, the more leadership he showed. He reminded me of when I was with the Jets and Joe Namath. Like Joe, he was a leader. When he was in the game, the players pass-blocked better, they made better catches, and they got those extra inches or runs. He had a tremendous capacity for leadership.

I've seen Brian continue to play after being severely hurt. Most other players would have been out of action a year, but Brian would be out for only ten minutes. I remember once in 1980, we were playing Green Bay a week after Brian had hurt his knee. The team doctor said, "Brian can play against Green Bay so long as he doesn't try to scramble out of the pocket." The Saturday morning before the game, Brian came to me and said, "Coach, I said yes to the doc so I could play, but you know I have to do what has to be done to win the game."

I said, "It's important that you take a sack if you see you're trapped. Don't get yourself hurt worse than you already are. You're the reason we're where we are in the division right now. Don't get hurt." We were in the middle of the race in 1980. The players had tremendous confidence in Brian and played hard. Early in the Green Bay game, Brian dropped back to pass and was chased out of the pocket. Instead of falling down for a sack, he ran behind Joe DeLamielleure and picked up 4 yards. Then I wanted him to run out of bounds so he wouldn't get hit, but he plowed ahead, holding onto the guard, and got an extra couple of yards.

In 1978, our first encounter with Cincinnati was the second game of the year. Everybody from Art Modell to the equipment men were nervous all week long. Boy, were they tight. That's when I realized just how important it was for Art to beat Paul Brown and the Bengals. We won that game 13–10 in overtime. When I went to Art's office, he was so excited it was like a Super Bowl win.

We went to Atlanta the next week and won. That made us 3–0. Next came Pittsburgh. They were also 3–0. At the end of four quarters we were tied 9–9. Three field goals each. No touchdowns. We lost the toss and kicked off to Pittsburgh to start the overtime. NFL has overtime to avoid ties. They fumbled the ball inside their own 20-yard line, and we recovered. I told Brian to go in with the offense. He turned to me and said, "Coach, they're not gonna give it to us." An official didn't acknowledge another official who had clearly seen the run-back fumble. We didn't get the ball. You talk about robbery! I couldn't believe that call. Nobody else could either. In that game, we had two touchdowns called back. Brian had hit Reggie Rucker and Tom Sullivan for touchdowns. Pittsburgh won. Mean Joe Greene said to me after the game, "If Gregg Pruitt hadn't been hurt and could have played for you today, we all would have gone home early." It was the beginning of a great rivalry between the two teams. Pittsburgh went on to win the Super Bowl in 1979 and 1980.

The year 1978 was a roller-coaster ride. We started 3–0, but by the eleventh game, we were 5–6, headed for Baltimore to play the Colts. Brian was struggling, and the press was hinting that "Sipe would be benched."

Before the game, Brian came to my office and said, "Coach, the most important thing for us to do is to win. I'm your quarterback. I'm the guy you can win with now and in the future."

I looked at Brian. He wasn't being cocky. He was simply confident. I said, "Brian, we made our commitment to you, and that's that. You're our quarterback. Don't pay any attention to the newspapers." We beat the Colts, and Brian had his first 300-yard passing game.

We ended up in Cincinnati 8–7 with a chance to get in the playoffs in our final game of the season. In the locker room at Cincinnati, Art Modell and Peter Hadhazy came to me before the game and presented me with a new five-year contract. It was a good thing it was before the game because Brian got hurt during the first series of downs and we lost, ending the season 8–8. I told Art after the game that I wouldn't hold him to the renewed contract if he wanted to take it back. He said, "No, Sam, you're a winner, and you're my guy for the future." I was elated for more than one reason. It immediately told the press and the players that Sam was going to be the coach for five more years. It gave me the kind of stability to build on for the future. But even with that renewed contract, I knew the truth of the statement, "You'd better win, baby. The future is now. It's not down the road."

While we were 5–6 that year, I remember going to Art Modell in his hotel room in Baltimore. I said, "Art, if we don't get the kind of personnel man we need to bring in good players, you'll eventually fire me."

# CHAPTER SEVENTEEN

# KARDIAC KIDS 1979

**W**e opened the 1979 season with an overtime win in New York. That summer we had made a big trade for Lyle Alzado, defensive end from the Denver Broncos. Bringing in Alzado told our players plenty about our intentions to build up the defense in a big way so we could get into the playoffs every year, which was our number-one goal. If you can do this, sooner or later you get into the Super Bowl.

Our second game that year was against Kansas City. In the final moments of the game, Brian Sipe threw a touchdown pass to Reggie Rucker, and we won it. The next week, Brian did the same thing in the final seconds of the game against the Colts. He threw a 75-yard pass to Ozzie Newsome deep in Colts territory. Then Don Cockroft kicked a field goal, and the Kardiac Kids were 3–0 for the year. Man, I loved it! What's even more important was that Art Modell loved it!

Next came the most important game we'd had in years. We were scheduled to play Dallas in Cleveland on "Monday Night Football." Live TV! The players were psyched up, and so was I. Both teams were undefeated. We had more than 80,000 at the game and 60 to 80 million people watching on television. Former President Gerald Ford was at the game as Art Modell's guest.

Brian Sipe's father came all the way from Hawaii to attend the game. He spent the entire week with Brian and came to practice every day. At the Dallas game, Brian's father saw his son bring the city of Cleveland to its feet, screaming for joy.

The city was starved for a winner. For years, Cleveland had been known as the dumping ground of baseball. The Cavaliers basketball team was struggling. The hockey team couldn't win and pulled out. All the frustrated energy of the city was focused on the Kardiac Kids.

111

We demolished the Dallas Cowboys that year. I told the players before the game in the locker room, "It's an opportunity of a lifetime to be involved in a game like this. It's gonna be a dogfight, and we know that it can literally come down to the very last play of the game. Regardless of what might happen, just hang in there together. And at the end of the day, we'll have taken one giant step——I'm dreamin' again——to Pasadena." Everybody yelled and cheered as I said, "OK, good luck, let's go!"

Our team played like a team possessed that night against Dallas. We used everything in our playbook. We changed our defenses to combat their blitz, and it worked. I can remember being on the sideline, yelling encouragement to Brian Sipe more than once, saying, "Great call! What a great call!" Brian killed them in the air, and our runners kept them off balance, beating them 26–7. Brian was brilliant that game against Dallas. The receivers were brilliant. Tom Darden intercepted a pass and ran for a touchdown. Roger Staubach hadn't thrown an interception in about 165 throws. We were on top of the world. Fans partied all night that night. But our victory had its price. We lost Dick Ambrose, Lyle Alzado, and Gregg Pruitt to injuries.

Then things changed. We lost the next three games. The vultures began to circle. They began to call our first four wins flukes, luck. Funny how quickly people change. Hero to heel in four easy weeks. The climb up the mountain is almost impossible, but the slide down is quick and easy. But our guys dug in and fired back. We won the next three in a row. But when we were 6–3, Gregg Pruitt went down, and we lost him for the year. That made us 7–3. Next, Jerry Sherk went down, and we lost him for the year. Jerry really never came back fully from his injuries after that.

The team played exciting football. We got the name Kardiac Kids because of all the last-minute drives that won our games. It was cliffhangers' heaven. My fingernails were short. They called us the "Good Guys," the guys with the white hats. Brian was throwing 300-yard games. In fact he threw eight touchdown passes against Pittsburgh in two games.

Brian was great, but so was Terry Bradshaw. They caught us at the end of regulation time, and we had to go to overtime. The ref tossed the coin to decide who would kick off and who would receive. Pittsburgh won the toss! They drove to field-goal range. I stood on the sideline where I felt helpless and limp. I yelled, "Miss it, miss it, miss it! Block that son-of-a-gun! Come on, baby! Block it, block it, block it! Come on, baby, one time, one time, baby, one time, one time, miss it!" With nine seconds left in overtime, they made the kick and beat us 33–30. It would be Pittsburgh who went to Pasadena, not us.

Inside the locker room, I said to the players, "Everybody get your head up. I couldn't be more proud of you. Hey, look, it was tough, and it was a hard-fought football game. You played the world's champions, and as I told you before the game, win, lose, or draw, you are all that matters to me. You just gotta take things like this, and you gotta grow. Now keep your heads up."

Brian Sipe's father had died on Wednesday prior to the Sunday game. Brian decided to play and leave for home in time for the funeral. I never experienced anything like the way the guys played their hearts out that day. We were overmatched in talent, but our guys had hearts that gave everything.

No one evaluates a coach properly. Just win, baby. The worst coach is a hero if he wins, but if Saint Christopher coached a losing team, he would be a bum. It's win or nothing. *No* coach or team can win them all every year. The true measure of a coach is how he maximizes the talent he has to work with. You have to have the horses to win the races.

After we lost to Pittsburgh, Brian came to my office just prior to leaving for his father's funeral in San Diego. Brian and I had talked many times, but that night was special. We talked of death and eternal life and the things that really matter when football is no longer a major consideration.

Our final game of the year was against Cincinnati. All we needed to do was win it, and we would be in the playoffs. It was a tough game. Cincinnati beat us, and we were out of the playoffs. All the talk and rationalization in the world wouldn't change the fact that Pittsburgh, not the Browns, went to the Super Bowl. Football is always a game of inches. The Kardiac Kids were in the toughest division in football, holding our own. But 8–8 and 9–7 wouldn't be good enough. We had to win more than that to be in the playoffs every year.

That year was one of the most exciting of my life. One person who helped keep it exciting was Lyle Alzado. Lyle was bigger than life almost all the time. He had a tremendous impact on our team. I had known Lyle because he came from Brooklyn originally. He played in Lawrence, Long Island, for a high school whose coach was Jack Martilotta, a good friend of mine. Denver drafted Lyle out of Yankton College in South Dakota after I left their coaching staff. In 1979, for some reason, they wanted to trade him.

Lyle, his agent, Art Modell, Peter Hadhazy, and I met secretly in Cleveland at Stouffer's Inn. Lyle was in town to see the Browns play that night against the Colts. He and I hit it off right away. Both from Brooklyn, right? Lyle and I were both street guys, and we understood each other. I knew somehow that Lyle was motivated by people who showed that they needed him. Big as he is, tough as he is, he's a human being with feelings just like anybody else.

I really liked the guy. Man, he was a player. The moment he felt you loved and needed him, he would do almost anything for you. He'd jump off the Brooklyn Bridge if you asked him to. He's what every football team needs. He controlled the pulse and the tempo of a game. He was often undisciplined, but he was 1950 dirt-tough. In the 1950s, players played more for fun than for profit. He truly loved the game. He was really a tough guy. He actually fought a fifteen-round exhibition fight against former World Champion Muhammad Ali at Mile Stadium in Denver. He was strong, though a bit undersized for an NFL tackle at six feet two and 250 pounds.

When he first came on our team, a lot of guys misinterpreted his motives. Lyle was simply a leader from the moment he arrived. Like all great leaders, he led by example. He danced every dance, never laid down, played hurt half the time, but never quit. He played from the time he arrived in the locker room until he returned there after the game. He gave the team the excitement and the kind of toughness that are really needed to win. He gave us those things in 1979, 1980, and 1981. Then I made a mistake.

Our defensive coaches told me they couldn't build a defense with Lyle Alzado because he was too undisciplined. I think it's very important to listen to your coaches, but the head coach had better make that kind of decision himself. I wanted to back up my coaches, but my heart wasn't in it. We traded Lyle to the Raiders where he had three or four great years, including a victory in the Super Bowl. In addition to that, he was selected for the Pro Bowl.

I blew it. They say a new broom sweeps clean, but it takes an old one to get in the corners. Lyle had the ingredient that every football player needs: toughness that's contagious. You just don't find that in every draft. In fact, you don't find it much at all anymore. Now players are astute businessmen with agents and endorsements and huge salaries and incentives. They don't seem to have the singleness of purpose that players used to have. Hey, I can't blame them, but the hoopla and the big money allow them to be less hungry when they play.

Of course Lyle had an agent and was interested in money, but he still played like a rookie who was trying to make the team. He simply loved to play football. You can say what you want about Lyle, and some other coaches and players wouldn't agree with me, but when old Lyle put his hand on the ground and the whistle blew, he played like a guy playing in 1940 or 1950 for twelve thousand bucks a year. He was hostile, he was excitable, he was vociferous. He was like a communicable disease. He spread his excitement in all directions within the team. That's what morale is all about. It can be bad or good, but it'll spread throughout your team, either way. When Lyle played the game, many of the other guys got fired up because he was. Sure, Lyle was known as a big mouth and he talked a lot, but he backed it up on the field. Joe Namath did the same thing. The difference was that Lyle screamed and scowled as he crushed his opponents while Broadway Joe smiled and picked the defense apart with his passes. But both those bigger-than-life guys were winners.

Lyle would do almost anything to win. Defensive linemen get paid to sack quarterbacks. They study their opposing offensive linemen all week and look for weaknesses to exploit. A defensive lineman tries to create a mismatch so he can defeat a blocker and get to the quarterback. In key third-down passing situations, the opposing linemen always expected Lyle to charge in the same way each time. Lyle knew they expected that too. The offensive tackles and support blockers on that side were assigned to block him. He loved to harass the opposition, to psyche them out.

Once during the game, Lyle went to the sideline and told another defensive end to "do a stunt" in the game. The other end said, "Hey, Lyle, I can't do that. Coach'll kill me!" Lyle shouted back, "Listen, you do it, and I'll take full responsibility." Lyle had his defensive teammate move quickly from the inside to Lyle's outside position. He then came down hard to the inside. The switch surprised the offensive linemen, and suddenly Lyle charged one on one toward a startled blocker who was no match for him. Lyle buried the quarterback. He had found a way to create a mismatch.

That time he succeeded, and so it was okay. He took a chance. If he had failed, he could have been a goat. Worse, the coaches would have really chewed him out. There just wasn't time to ask the coaches. Lyle was a veteran who had the moxie to spot a weakness, and he went for it.

We had all of that on tape on the sideline, and it was in the NFL high-lights film the next year. It was something Lyle thought up that he certainly should have discussed with the coach, but in the heat of the game Lyle didn't think there would be time for talk. It wasn't in the game plan, of course, but it worked very well. Now it's preserved on tape as a brilliant football move. Most coaches would put a stop to things like that, but sometimes you have to give a thoroughbred his head.

At other times, he would drive you crazy with his emotional out-bursts. Sometimes he would come into the locker room at halftime and ram his fist through a locker door. Sometimes he would pick up a chair and fling it the length of the locker room. Once he came into the locker room and spotted a big stack of fruit on a table that had been prepared for the players. He was so mad that he shoved all the fruit onto the floor, and he used all the bad language known to man and some extra thrown in while he was doing it. During the games, he gave so much of himself that the other players followed his lead. The trick was to teach them to follow his good examples, not his bad ones. But you can't ex-pect a player to be a lion on the field and a lamb in the locker room. Besides, boys will be boys!

In 1979 when we lost to Pittsburgh 33-30 in Pittsburgh, it was simply unacceptable to Lyle. Other players handled the loss differently, and some hated the way Lyle handled it. Even in practice, if Lyle thought guys were dogging it, he would curse them out loud and say, "You guys don't want to work, you don't want to win." Somebody would get mad and answer, "Why don't you shut up, you phony?" Lyle would strip his helmet off and charge over to the other guy, and we'd have to break up a fight. Although you hate to see things like that happen, it does show the intensity of Lyle's spirit and will to win. It had its effect on the players, no question about it. Even the ones who didn't like him played a little harder because of him. Hey, football is a very emotional game, and it's played from the neck up. It's an emotional game played in the real estate between your ears. People talk about all the physical aspects of football, but emotion is what it's all about. You have to play emotion-ally but under control. Lyle lost control once in a while. You can't man-ufacture emotion; it must come from within.

Doug Dieken, on the other hand, was as tough as Lyle Alzado, but he was very quiet and controlled. Some would say the difference was between sanity and insanity. Doug was a finesse guy who played cerebrally. He didn't have the physical toughness that Lyle had, but somehow he was just as tough. Doug was only the third left tackle in the history of the Cleveland Browns. Lou Groza and Dick Schafrath preceded him in that position. Doug broke everybody's record in consistent games played.

The Kardiac Kids were a special group of athletes. They all were overachievers who played up to their maximum each week. Coaches are rarely so privileged to be around a group of players who can reach their potential and play that way week in and week out.

# CHAPTER EIGHTEEN

# 1980 KARDIAC KIDS AGAIN

**W**e opened the 1980 season hailed as the Kardiac Kids again. Expectations were high. Everybody thought we would take up where we left off last season. When we lost our first game to New England at their stadium, I was really depressed.

A "Monday Night Football" televised game against Houston at our stadium was coming up the next week. With our fans behind us, we were sure to win it. All the screaming and yelling helped during the game, but it wasn't enough to ensure a win. Down two in a row and the season was just starting. Already I had a lot of anxiety about facing Art Modell. But I couldn't run, and I couldn't hide. No obedient child wanted to please his father more than I wanted to win for Art Modell.

I went up to the office after the game. Art and Peter Hadhazy were as blue as my shirt. They had really counted on a continuation of our improvement in 1979. In 1978 we were 8–8. We were 9–7 in 1979. In 1980 they wanted more, of course. They felt we would simply take off in 1980 and go all the way to the Super Bowl. We won eleven of the next fourteen games, and the Kardiac Kids were back in business. But we did lose a crucial game to Denver, and we lost in the final plays of our games against Pittsburgh and Minnesota. We very easily could have won thirteen or fourteen games. As I've said before, football is a game of inches, and twelve of the sixteen games we played that year were decided in the final two minutes.

Things happened in Cleveland that were very different to me. I heard Christmas songs with my name in them. The hype was unbelievable. The city was really stirred up by its football team. The one thing I prayed a lot about was that I didn't really know who the head coach of the Browns was. I knew who Sam Rutigliano was, but this coach I kept reading about was a mystery to me. All the attention I received was new to me. I had been with losing teams for eleven years. Now I was king of the hill and Coach of the Year for the second consecutive year. I prayed hard that I would be able to keep my perspective. I may not have known who the head coach of the Browns was, but I knew who *I* was. That was very important to me.

The most incredible game of the year was the fifteenth one. When we went to Minnesota, we were 10–4. If we beat them, we would be the only AFC team to qualify for the playoffs in game fifteen. I can still see it so plainly in my mind. We've got the game won with sixteen seconds to go. Minnesota is on their own 20-yard line with no more time-outs. They throw a pass to the tight end who laterals to the fullback, Ted Brown. If we tackle this man now, the game is over and we win. He sidesteps a tackler and runs out of bounds on the 50-yard line. We know then that Tommy Kramer, the quarterback, is going to throw a desperation pass into the end zone. We defend in two levels with Tom Darden as our free safety. We tell Tom to jump up and swat the ball out of bounds but, above all, not to swat it down. The teams line up against each other. This game is in the bag for us. There's no way they can go 80 yards in sixteen seconds with no time-outs. Already I'm anticipating the jubilation in the locker room. Already I'm smiling inside as I picture the press conference. I'm especially anxious to see Art's joy. I loved to see that guy joyful. Sometimes I felt that was my main assignment as a head coach—to make the owner joyful and happy. There was one way and only one way to do that: win, baby!

The ball is snapped. Kramer fades back into the pocket and hangs the desperation pass up, up in the sky. I'm running along the sideline on my tiptoes, almost trying to tip the pass away myself. I'm screaming to Tom Darden, "Knock it down! Knock it down! Swat it into the bleachers! Get up there! Jump! Jump up, up, up!" I watch as Darden goes up, just as we told him to. "Great, Tom's got it, he's got it! Knock it out of bounds, Tom!" Then I can't believe my eyes. It can't be! He tips the ball up in the air, just as we told him not to, right into Ahmad Rashad's hands for the reception. "Oh, no! I can't believe it! He tipped it up, he tipped it up!" I'm numb. Merry Christmas, Ahmad Rashad! Here's a gift for you! It'll be on the NFL highlights film for years. Ahmad falls into the end zone for a touchdown. We lose. Minnesota wins their division. They're going to the playoffs. Our team is devastated.

In sixteen short seconds we went from the thrill of victory to the agony of defeat. The people in the stands went crazy. It was total bedlam on the field. The referee ran up to me and said, "You gotta get eleven guys on the field for the extra point try."

"You're outta your mind! You'd be better off trying to get eleven people outta the stands than my guys. The game's over." I trotted off the field and into the locker room.

What could I say to my players? They were wiped out. Anything I said would be a lame attempt. I wanted to fall in a hole and hide. One of the biggest challenges for a football coach is when he has to follow his players into the locker room after a defeat. That's when he really earns his money. The players have to be picked back up. The coach must help them pull their tails back up off the ground. Some of them hang their heads, some of them slam their helmets to the floor, some of them kick the lockers, some of them slam their forearms against the wall. They have to do something to vent their disappointment and frustration. I couldn't find a hole to hide in. Besides, they were all looking to me for direction. I really knew how they felt. I had been there as a player. In a situation like this the head coach, alone, must convince the players to put this one behind them and get ready for the Cincinnati game next week.

When you face those players after a loss, you don't get any feeling of encouragement from them at all. They just slump in the chairs by their lockers. It's like going door-to-door trying to sell refrigerators to Eskimos. It's tough.

The first thing I did was to clear the locker room of everyone but players and staff. I gathered the players in a circle and asked them to face me. I stood where all of them could see me. I told them to look at me and listen good because I was going to speak only five minutes. I wanted all of us to have eye contact. These guys were athletes who had listened to the likes of Joe Paterno at Penn State, Bear Bryant at Alabama, and Bo Schembeckler at Michigan. They had heard it all. Still I had to tell them something, and if I wasn't careful, they would turn me off. I said, "Through trials and tribulations you have to persevere. Perseverance gives character and character gives hope. We lost a battle, but we can still win the war next week." A coach must know the right thing to say in critical situations, or he can lose his team. How often I thought of my father's advice: "If you have an opportunity to keep your mouth shut, take advantage of it. You make many mistakes in the things you say, but rarely do you make a mistake in your silence."

Red Auerbach said it best when he said, "The definition of over-coaching is when a coach falls in love with the sound of his own voice." We all fall into that trap once in a while as we communicate. There is no key. You must have the feeling for a situation in order to respond. The players needed me, and the best way to get them back on track was to give them a pat on the back. In coaching football you must wait a week between games, but in baseball you come back the next day and play. It means you get more deeply involved in the psychology of human behavior in football because of the time lapse between games.

What we did to the New York Jets in 1979, Minnesota did to us in 1980. We just didn't make the play that we should have, but Minnesota did. That's football. Our world was turned upside down in sixteen seconds.

When I got on the bus, Art Modell and Peter Hadhazy looked like they had just written suicide notes and they were going to take their lives. They couldn't look me in the eye. They had hired this guy, Sam Who, and now everybody knew my name and could even pronounce it correctly. I felt like Benedict Arnold. I had taken their team to game fifteen in which a win would have put us in the playoffs, and we lost it. We could have been flying back to Cleveland right then worried about the size of the crowd waiting for us at the airport.

Our next game, which was the last of the season, was with Cincinnati at their stadium. We had lost to Cincinatti in 1978 and 1979 in the last games of those years. I sat there thinking, *This year they're 6–9. We should kill them. They're disorganized. They fired their coach. Forrest Gregg is their new head coach. He hasn't had time to regroup his players. We should stomp them good.*

But Art Modell's team was going up against two guys he fired: Paul Brown and Forrest Gregg. Because of our last two losses to Cincinnati, we were under even more pressure than usual. You never take anything for granted. You never know what's going to happen in football. Our going to Cincinnati was like a bear raiding a hornet's nest. There would be plenty of action.

The memories moved in on me again as we approached the game. I remembered Blanton Collier, who took over for Paul Brown after the latter was fired by Art Modell. When I first came to Cleveland, Blanton was retired. He said to me, "Being a head coach in the National Football League is the loneliest job in the world. There will be times when you will have absolutely no one to talk to, not even your wife and certainly not the owner." (I can identify with Paul Brown's feelings because he, too, was fired by Art Modell.) More than anyone, Blanton knew what was going on in Art Modell's mind and Paul Brown's mind during those great Browns-Bengals games that I coached.

Blanton always encouraged me during those times by writing me letters just prior to each game. He knew exactly how I felt facing those special games. He wanted me to know that, win or lose, he was in my back pocket. The thrill of victory and the agony of defeat were intensified in those Browns-Bengals games. Not only did Paul Brown want to win those games, he wanted to blow us out of the stadium.

Now here we were in 1980 playing the final game of the season. We had lost in the final games of 1978 and 1979, but now the stakes were higher. We needed to win this game, not only to win the division, but to qualify for the playoffs.

Art Modell was a basket case all week long. I changed our routine and cut down on our meetings and practice sessions. I told the team not to get involved in all the ifs and buts and candy and nuts that everybody else was talking about. I said, "Let's just concentrate on our jobs. Let's not get into the game of coulda, woulda, and shoulda."

On the bus on the way to the Cincinnati stadium, I sat down in my usual seat while Art and Pat Modell sat down in their usual seat. Art got up, came over, and sat down beside me, "Listen, Sam, no matter what happens today, we'll still be 10–6 and everybody'll be excited. You've had a great year."

I said, "Art, You're fulla baloney! You wanta win this game more than you wanta breathe. It's really gonna be a tough game, but I think we're gonna win it." Art laughed.

That game, like all tough games, still lives in my memory. I think about it sometimes at night just before I go to sleep. We're 10–10 at the half. When the second half starts, Brian Sipe throws an interception for a touchdown. He trots over to me at the sideline and says, "Listen, Coach, we're gonna win this game. There's no way in the world we're gonna lose it."

"Brian, I believe you because you've pulled it off so many times before." I smiled at him and said, "But you gotta promise to start throwing the ball to *our* guys!"

I remembered then the scene in the locker room just before the game. I had said everything a coach can say, and they were about ready to run out on the field. Then I looked at them and said, "Look men, there're 800 million Chinese who won't care if we win or lose today." I wanted to loosen them up. Boy, were they tight. The veterans started to laugh, and then the young players started to laugh after the veterans led the way. I wanted to get the nervousness out of them. I wanted to give them the proper perspective. Later the news media picked up my "Chinese" statement out of context and had a field day with it. I wanted the players to go out there and express their talents and not have a grapefruit in their esophagus. But the press made it sound as if I didn't care if we won or lost. Some of those guys should write fiction for a living. Bobby Knight might be right when he says, "We all learn to read and write at an early age and then go on to bigger and better things."

I can still see it in my mind. The game flows back and forth, and we just can't run the football. I'm screaming at the guys, "Protect Brian, you guys, circle the wagons around him! Cut those pass rushers down. Come on!" We had protected our quarterback better than any other NFL team all season. Proof of the pudding was that Jo DeLamielleure, Tom DeLeone, and Doug Dieken were all going to the Pro Bowl. Brian Sipe had already been named the starting quarterback for the Pro Bowl. Mike Pruitt was going to the Pro Bowl. We had five offensive players selected to play in the Pro Bowl. Pass protection is the most important element in passing situations. You have to build a barbed-wire fence around your quarterback. Cincinnati was like a sleeping giant to us. I had told our players all week long, "Don't wake this giant up." So what happens?

By now Cincinnati is so fired up they sack Sipe six times. He throws two interceptions. We can't run the football. Cincinnati wants our blood. To them, this game *is* the Super Bowl. I'm thinking, *If they can stop us, Paul Brown will probably give Forrest Gregg a new ten-year contract on the spot! Oh, how they want to win this game. Even with their bad season, knocking us out of the playoffs will make it all worthwhile to them.*

The clock ticks down to the final minutes of the game. We hold them in three downs, and they have to kick. Their kicker, Paul McInally, shanks the ball out of bounds. I wave my arms in the air and yell to the guys, "OK, you guys, this is the break we've been waiting for! Get in there and do it!" Football is a game of field position. We have excellent position at midfield. A couple of first downs and we can kick a field goal.

We get the ball on the 50-yard line. Great field position. The score is now 24–24 with two minutes left in the game. We keep pounding away, and suddenly our running game opens up. Defenses get tired late in the game. You have to be patient, like a fighter waiting for his opponent to drop his guard. When a guy like Mike Pruitt keeps pounding away at the line, he's going to cause some soft spots eventually.

We get down in their territory. I tell Sipe to eat up the clock. Nobody is any better at doing that than Brian. He hands off here, throws a short pass there, and now we're in field-goal position. We've got another down. Do we try to get closer, or do we try the field goal now? Many a coach has had to make that decision. Many a coach has been second-guessed for years because of such decisions. Coaches get fired and hired because of those decisions. Now I've got to make that decision. I decide to go for the field goal. It's a nervous situation. You don't want to take any chances, right?

With less than a minute to go, Don Cockcroft trots onto the field. They line up. I can hardly stand the wait. It's only seconds, but it seems like forever. I yell to Cockcroft, to the players all around me, to the heavens, "Make it good! It's just a chip shot, Don! You can do it!" He lunges forward. I hold my breath. "Make it, make it, make it, make it, make it!" His foot hits the ball. I watch it sail up high. "Be there, ball, be there! Hey, he's got it, it's gonna make it. He's got it, he's got it! All *right!*" What a beautiful sight, straight and true through the uprights! "I love it! Good shot, Don!" We're ahead 27–24, with less than a minute to go. It looks like a winner. But with Cincinnati it's never over till it's over.

We kick off to Cincinnati. They're out of time-outs. We have to keep them in bounds to keep the clock running. They complete a pass and Ron Bolton makes the tackle, but they're in field-goal range. Not again! Not three years in a row! I can't believe it's about to happen again! The clock is still running. Just a few seconds left. I'm screaming, "Block it, block it, block it! Kill it! Stop um!" The clock shows no time left, but their players are still scrambling to line up. "Is it over? Is the game over? Hey, Ref, is the game over, or isn't it, for cryin' out loud? Hey, somebody, anybody, is the game over? Hey stop them. They can't line up! Time has run out. Hey, Ref!" *God, don't let anything stupid happen this time!* It's not over till the fat lady stops singing! "Hey, did anybody hear the whistle? I didn't hear the whistle! Watch it, you guys!"

Finally it sinks in that the game is over. The Bengals couldn't line up in time. I let a big breath of relief out, which is better than taking Rolaids. Our players are jumping up on the sideline and hugging and slapping high fives all over the place. When the finality of it hit me, I could have even kissed Lyle Alzado! Boy, boy, joy, joy! Browns win it, 27–24!

Reggie Rucker and Lyle Alzado grab me and carry me off the field. In the locker room it's bedlam. TV, radio, and press people are everywhere. Players are jumping up and down. Art Modell is hugging everybody and clapping his hands. All the management people are there. We win the division, the very best division in professional football. Everybody loves a winner. We had come a long, long way in three years against tremendous odds.

After a few minutes, I sat the players down and we prayed, right on national television. After the prayer, I gathered the players around me and said, "These are the moments to savor. You'll remember this day the rest of your life. Enjoy it. Get a still-shot of it in your mind so you can picture it later. You're on the mountaintop now. Enjoy it because for every peak there's a valley. This is your moment to remember always. You did it. You won this game. You may never again have a moment as sweet as this one, so bask in it now. Thanks for a super win." Then the guys went back to celebrating, and the locker room was a noisy, happy place.

Such a big win brings out the very best in everybody. Deep emotions come out of people who are usually reserved. Chills slice through your body like electric knives. I look around and grin at the sight of Dick Ambrose yelling happily at his teammates. Dick hardly ever says a word. Sweet victory. I watch Calvin Hill, a number-one draft choice of the Dallas Cowboys and a Yale graduate.

I see right here in the locker room that football is a microcosm of society. It's the one time, between the boundaries of that field measuring one hundred yards long and fifty-three and a third yards wide, that twenty-two players have a chance for glory. It doesn't matter if the owner is Jewish and the head coach is Italian, or if the white quarterback is from San Diego and the black fullback is from Chicago. On the field no one really cares where anybody comes from or who they are.

It's one of the things I always enjoyed as a coach. All of us were on the mountaintop together after winning a big game. We didn't need liquor or champagne in the locker room. Everybody was high from the win. Each of us knew how far we'd come since training camp. It was like climbing a sand hill. At the beginning of the year we took ten steps forward and slid back five steps. We were able to regroup, and now we were flipping out with joy. But you can't trust locker rooms. Just four short years later I would be in the same locker room waiting for my Armageddon.

When we landed at Cleveland, 25,000 people were waiting to greet us. It was like the Crusaders coming home after a victorious battle. The terminal was so crowded we couldn't go in. They got special buses for us and unloaded out on the landing field. Mayor Voinovich was there. They finally got us organized, and all the players were introduced on a flatbed truck. It was an unforgettable experience. We were going to play the first playoff game in Cleveland since 1972.

After Art and Pat and I got to their house, I called Barb and told her to join us there. Blanton Collier called from Houston, Texas, to congratulate us. It was an exhilarating time. It was like Mardi Gras, Christmas, and New Year's Eve all on the same day. What a joyous time to be able to share together. Art was not just the owner I coached for; he was, by then, my friend. It was pure fun for us to be together at times like that. If only it could last.

It's difficult to describe how a coach feels about his owner. The owner doesn't coach or draft the players. He sits up in the loge during the games and doesn't have moment-by-moment contact. Contrary to what some people think, Art never tried to call the game from his box. He never interfered with the coaching staff that way. I used to enjoy so much seeing Art and Pat during the bus rides, the plane rides, and in their home after the games. It was such a tremendous feeling to share with an owner who had a great sense of humor and who offered such great togetherness. I didn't want the day to end. But, through it all, there was always that little shadow in the back of my mind. The Cincinnati victory was one of the sweetest, but there would always be another game.

Barb and I continued our celebration with the kids at our own home later that night. It was Fantasy Land. It's a dream and you don't want to wake up.

I spent the next day with the players. We didn't do anything except celebrate. We didn't even look at the game film. We gave the players the rest of the week off. They deserved it. Then we would open up next week with practice in preparation for the playoff opener at our stadium against the Oakland Raiders. It was going to be a war.

# CHAPTER NINETEEN

# I WAS BORN AT NIGHT, BUT NOT LAST NIGHT

**W**e were 8–8 in 1978, 9–7 in 1979, and 11–5 in 1980. We were very happy with our steady improvement. I was Coach of the Year in 1979 and 1980. I was enthused and optimistic at the beginning of 1981. So were the football fans of Cleveland. We started off the year with two losses. Then we won two. We lost two more, which meant we were 2–4. We won the next two. Because we had come from behind twice, we felt we could really go for the drive during the rest of the season. It wasn't to be. We won only one out of the next eight games. Ironically, the games we won in 1980, we lost the same way in 1981.

Everything happened that year. During training camp, Rich Kotite, who is now the offensive coordinator for the New York Jets, came to see me in my office one day. He told me he was having severe headaches and blurred vision. That summer he had seen a doctor who told him it was hypertension. Rich was very concerned. He made an appointment with a neurologist at the Cleveland Clinic that very afternoon. Later that afternoon, one of our coaches got a call from Rich's wife, Liz, who was in New York City. She said Rich had just called her from a telephone booth and he was very upset. The doctors had discovered a large mass in his head. She said Rich was terrified. The doctors didn't know if it was malignant or not. Barb and I went to visit Rich that night at the clinic. As I looked at Rich in his state of fear, I realized that getting to the Super Bowl is not always the most important thing in the world. This man was waiting for news that could mean the end of his life. The number-one priority in my life for those moments was to be with Rich Kotite.

In a few hours, we learned that the pituitary tumor was probably benign. Rich's operation lasted nine and a half hours and was a complete success. Seventeen days later, when we played our opening game on "Monday Night Football" against San Diego, Rich was at work in the press box and on the field wearing a baseball helmet. Barb just shook her head and said, "Only in football! If anybody else had a brain tumor operation, he would be off work for six to nine months."

The only highlights of that year were our victories over Cincinnati and San Francisco. That was the season San Francisco beat Cincinnati in the Super Bowl. It was a tough year for everybody. In 1980, Sipe was able to pull off wins in the last seconds of many games. But in 1981, we were losing many games in the last seconds. It didn't make any sense to me.

Toward the end of the year, we played Houston at Houston on national television on a Thursday night. We were at the end of the game, we were down inside the 5-yard down, and Brian Sipe actually thought it was third down. He called a draw play, and Cleo Miller was tackled short of the goal line, and the game was over. Nobody could believe what had happened. Brian simply lost count. That was our fourth down. How could we go from eleven wins last season to five wins this season?

It was a mystery to me. I thought long and hard about it. I just couldn't make sense out of what was happening. Some of the players were dogging it. I didn't put two and two together until I got a telephone call from Carl Eller in the spring of 1982. He had just been released from a detoxification center in Phoenix, Arizona. Carl had played pro ball for over thirteen years, he went to four Super Bowls and five Pro Bowls, and he probably will be a Hall of Famer. He was one of the finest defensive ends who ever played the game. I didn't know Carl personally. All I knew was that when we played Minnesota, we could never block the left end, Number 81, Carl Eller.

Carl called right out of the blue. He said, "Coach, I'm a recovering drug addict. There's a huge problem in the National Football League with drugs. Nobody seems to be aware of it, and nobody wants to talk about it. I can tell you it's a big problem. I'm trying to talk to any of the teams who will listen to me. Not everybody wants to hear what I have to say. I'd like to talk to your players if you want me to. I'd like to give you an earful. It's unbelievable what's going on. I want to help as many young players as I can before it's too late for them."

"Gee, Carl, I'm flattered that you would call me. I'm sure you can talk with our players, but we don't have a drug problem."

Silence on the other end of the phone. Presently Carl said, "Whattaya say, Coach, do you want me to talk to your guys?"

"Hey listen, Carl, it wouldn't hurt, even if we don't have a problem. I'm sure the guys would want to listen to you anyway, you're such a legend."

So Carl came to Cleveland and talked with me, our staff, and our team. He told us how to watch for symptoms in the players. Then I began to think about all those losses in 1981. Wow, maybe some of our guys were on drugs. It began to make sense, but I didn't want to believe it.

I had to get to the bottom of this. How blind could I get? I felt like any father who first hears about drugs in his neighborhood. "Yeah, I know there's a problem out there, but not with *my* kids." Carl Eller had begun to open my eyes. I had to know more before I could say anything to Art Modell. I still found it hard to believe that our football team had any kind of drug problem.

Carl was not in any way suggesting that there was a problem on our team. He was giving his message to any and all who would listen. He said there were a lot of ostriches in the NFL who had their heads buried in the sand. He had gone through a period of thirteen years in which he had graduated from alcohol to marijuana to cocaine to supporting a habit costing $3,000 to $4,000 per week. He lost his wife, over $2 million, and almost his life. During the time he was a player and a user, he had a great fear of being discovered. He didn't want to be a user, but he was hooked. He was afraid he would be kicked out of the league if he came forward and confessed that he was a user. Because he was such a great player, he was able to keep going all the time he was a user. He said it was sad to think of how much better he could have been if he had been clean. Carl said drugs never improved his performance; they only improved his desire to use drugs.

Because of Carl's influence, we trained our coaches to be able to spot users. Carl gave us a list of things to watch out for. Denying use, pathological lying, being late for meetings, sleeping in meetings, missing airplane flights, not participating in a meeting—all were clues. We began watching the players on film to spot inconsistencies. We brought specialists in to talk to our players about alcohol and chemical dependency. The league office said every team should have a local psychiatrist who was a chemical dependency specialist. That's when we located a doctor. Even with all this activity and education, I believed it was all preventative, not curative. I just couldn't believe we had any drug users on our team.

But after we got educated, we did notice the symptoms, clues we were blind to before. We began comparing notes. Soon a pattern began to emerge, which made it obvious to anyone who was interested enough to watch. I told all the coaches to monitor the players and report back.

Our eyes started to open wider and wider in 1982. A coach would report, "Hey, this guy is sleeping in meetings." Another would say, "This guy is just making it to practice in the nick of time every day. He always used to be punctual." Management could watch for the big financial problems. "This guy is having highs and lows, and he used to be pretty stable." "This guy seems to be an altogether different person from what he used to be." "This guy has become more and more belligerent." "This guy isn't a reckless player anymore. He's not throwing his body all over the place like he used to. He's not playing as alert as he did before. He's not passing his written tests in the meetings."

Drug use increases desire, not performance. I remember players who in previous years were positive, coachable, and responsive. After becoming users, they were surly, negative and, in some cases, belligerent, particularly in training camp as they responded to injuries. In football, if you're injured, you don't play, but if you're hurting, you play. It's all part of the game. No gain without pain.

One player had always been tough and had played with the little hurts most players have, but suddenly he seemed to have made an about-face. He became belligerent about wanting to skip practice one Friday, even though the trainer said he was all right. I was surprised, but I brushed it aside as a normal mood swing.

As we became more educated, we responded more intelligently to such mood swings if they became behavior patterns. We alerted all the employees to be on the lookout for players who seemed to be in some kind of trouble. I told the staff it wasn't necessary to report to me every day. I told them to build up a list. I told them not to preach or moralize to the players, not to diagnose because we're not qualified to do those types of evaluations. It was our job to spot the symptoms we had been overlooking because we weren't trained before Carl Eller came on the scene. The one big thing I realized about users was how adept they became at deception.

We brought all kinds of professionals in to talk to the players, to tell them how drugs were "demons of deception," which only caused them to *feel* as if they were performing well. Since there are people around who would love to see marijuana legalized, many of the players were confused. I think the whole idea of legalization is preposterous. Only losers believe that drugs won't hurt you. Even some doctors are in favor of legalizing marijuana. They're absolutely wrong because that's how the entire thing starts with drugs.

It was through our program of intervention, prevention, and education that we were able to go from being naive to becoming street-smart. We were able to recognize suspicious actions of the players. Still, I believed our efforts would be more preventative than curative. *After all, we didn't have a problem on our team,* I thought.

Our drug education was a painful eye-opener. We learned that the average age of children who experiment with drugs or alcohol is 11.7 years. The easiest legal drug to obtain is alcohol. Approximately 3.3 million problem drinkers in the United States are between the ages of 14 and 17. Alcohol contributes to 50 percent of all our highway fatalities. The easiest illegal drug to obtain is marijuana. There are many reasons why it is considered to be the most threatening drug to adolescents. It gives a quick "high." They believe it to be safe. It's readily available, and there are no immediate withdrawal symptoms such as hangovers. Today marijuana is five to ten times stronger than it was just a few years ago. One joint of marijuana will leave traces of the drug in the body from seven to thirty days. Marijuana causes psychological addiction, and it can lead to physical addiction.

I knew these statistics were widely known. I knew they didn't compare to all the deaths each year on American highways. We've had more deaths on our highways than the total of all deaths in all our wars. Statistics and slogans won't dissuade people from using drugs. The problem in our society is that we are in a very real war against alcohol, drugs, and chemical dependency. We aren't prepared or mobilized to fight against this war. I believe that most people in America are not aware that we're involved in a war. Many parents of today came out of the 1960s. Now their children are in school. We very well could lose a generation because of our apathy toward drugs.

I'm reminded of a man who was standing by a river. Suddenly, he saw two people thrashing in the water, close to drowning, as they floated downstream. The man wasn't a very good swimmer, but he plunged in and managed to save the two people. When he pulled them ashore, he stood there exhausted, trying to recover his breath. He noticed a man standing there watching but not making any effort to help. Then he noticed another man struggling in the water, and he dived in and swam out to him. The panic-stricken man grabbed his rescuer and dragged him under. With superhuman effort, the swimmer managed to pull the man ashore, saving his life. He noticed with dismay that the man watching on shore hadn't moved. The rescuer yelled at the observer, "Hey, you see what's going on here. Why don't you help me? I've almost drowned myself!" The man answered, "I'm not going to help you. I'm going upriver to find out who's throwing them in."

That little story gives an idea of what's going on today in the drug scene. We're involved in a lot of things of a curative nature, and we're sidetracked by legalities. We're arguing about the Fourth Amendment to the Constitution, the invasion of privacy, and random drug testing while somebody upstream is gleefully free to throw in more and more bodies. Professional football, baseball, and basketball have drug programs. But now they have to have a collective bargaining agreement with the unions.

People are *talking* a lot about drugs. Meantime, we've got more young people who are committing suicide in the USA than in the history of the world. We need to get all the prevailing minds together and begin to *do* something positive. One person I know of who is doing a good job is Dr. Richard Dobbins of Emerge Ministries in Akron, Ohio. He said it best, "Until the pain of remaining the same hurts more than the pain to change, people prefer to remain the same."

We're at that point now where it really hurts more to stay the same. In the sports world some athletes are choosing to abstain from drugs, but many others aren't. Two star athletes died in quick succession by making the wrong choices: Len Bias, the basketball player for the University of Maryland who was drafted by the Boston Celtics as the second player in the NBA draft, and Don Rogers, the first-draft choice All-American chosen by the Cleveland Browns. Both of these outstanding young athletes died of an overdose of cocaine. If it's "good medicine" and not an "invasion of privacy" to vaccinate every young person in America against disease, why isn't it equally good medicine and no more of an invasion of privacy to have mandatory drug testing? If mandatory drug testing is not allowed, then won't someone soon push for legislation to stop vaccinations on the same grounds?

We didn't know it when we started our "prevention" program, but the dam was about to break all around us.

# CHAPTER TWENTY

# SEEDS WERE PLANTED

The first playoff game was in January 1981 in Cleveland Municipal Stadium against the Oakland Raiders. The temperature was below zero. The windchill factor was minus twenty-nine degrees. It was absolutely unbelievable. I have never seen playing conditions so bad. Football has so much contact and takes about three and a half hours for a complete game. I saw players take off their gloves only to find frozen perspiration beneath their fingernails. I saw black players whose black beards and mustaches were crusted with silver ice.

I had never been bothered by the weather simply because the excitement and my movements on the sideline always kept me warm. The adrenaline runs fast. But this game was different. There was no way to keep warm. My ears felt like they would fall off. The arctic air stung my chest as I inhaled. The collective steam from all our breathing looked like a scene out of Doctor Zhivago.

Almost all the advantages and abilities of the skilled players were neutralized. People like Dave Logan, Ozzie Newsome, Reggie Rucker, Gregg Pruitt, Mike Pruitt, and Brian Sipe were reduced to being average performers in weather conditions as severe as we had. On the other hand, the defense couldn't rush the passer very well, but neither could the offense dig in and run. I remember one end-zone play where Reggie Rucker caught a pass out of the end zone and couldn't stop running because of the ice. He slipped and slid all the way into the dugout. I remember it like it happened yesterday.

The game is going back and forth, and both teams are waiting for a break. We're losing 14–12 in the closing minutes of the fourth quarter. The Raiders are driving for a touchdown or a field goal. They're killing the clock. It's their fourth down, and they have less than the length of a football to go for a first down. Now Tom Flores, the head coach of the

133

Raiders, has to make a decision. If he makes the first down, we have to call our last time-out, he kills the clock and kicks a field goal, and the game is over. He goes for the first down. I would have called the same play. Who couldn't gain a few inches? Any team that couldn't do that didn't deserve a first down, right? A first down could win the game. They snap the ball. The lines surge. Dick Ambrose and Robert L. Jackson make one of the greatest plays I've ever seen. Their fullback, Mark van Eeghen, is carrying the ball. He *always* picks up short yardage. I'll guarantee you, if he tries it one thousand times, you can bet the house, the mortgage, the ranch, he is gonna make four inches! No way is he *not* gonna make it. Blam! We stop him.

Brian Sipe comes to the sideline to talk. I tell him to pass, pass, pass. He goes back in, and he's like Superman. Faster than a speeding bullet, he throws a pass to Reggie Rucker, then another one to Ozzie Newsome, then one to Gregg Pruitt. Now it's first down on their 13-yard line with a minute and thirty-five seconds left in the game. We've moved the ball from inside our own 15-yard line to their 13! We call time-out. All we have to do is kick a field goal, and the game is over.

We talk it over on the sideline again. Our kicker has already missed 1 extra point and three field goals. What do you do as a coach? You go with what has been working for you all during the game, right? We know any field-goal attempt is not going to be a routine chip shot, not in this weather. Our strategy is to run the ball on our first and third downs to keep the clock running. If they call a time-out on the third down, they have no more time-outs. Then we'll kick the field goal and go ahead. When we kick off to them, they'll have less than a minute to go with no more time-outs, and they'll have to drive from deep in their own territory. Not bad odds under these conditions.

We run the ball on first down, and the clock keeps running. We decide to throw the ball on second down. If we throw an incompletion on second down, we still have a third down to get the clock running again. So we come up with a set play. Ozzie Newsome is to go down the middle, Reggie Rucker is to go from right to left, and Dave Logan is to be on the weakest corner. Lester Hayes, an All-Pro cornerback, would be all over Reggie Rucker. We keep Pruitt in to block so that Sipe won't have to worry about his left side. For a right-handed quarterback, the left side is the blind side. We can't afford a sack or an interception.

I say to Brian, "If the situation gets tight, if the defense looks like Times Square on New Year's Eve, if you feel at all that you have to force the ball, throw it into Lake Erie, throw it into some blonde's lap in the bleachers, but *don't* throw the ball into the middle of the field."

Brian drops back to pass, and our play develops beautifully, just as we anticipated. Rucker is smothered by Hayes as we anticipated, Ozzie is going straight ahead, and here comes Dave Logan from left to right—wide open for a touchdown. I'm already celebrating. It's so beautiful to see one of your plays develop and work right in front of your eyes. The joy is pouring up from my gut; I can't stop it. Just a little 10-yard toss, Brian, and it's in the bag. Toss it to Dave, Brian! I have no doubt in the world that Brian will throw the ball to Dave, that Dave will catch it and step into the end zone for a touchdown and a win. The play, a crossing pattern versus man-to-man coverage, is designed for Dave Logan. I can already taste the victory. "Hit Dave, Brian, he's wide open!" I yell and run along the sideline. "Hit 'im, Brian!" One little 10-yard pass, Brian, and we're on our way to San Diego to play in the championship game and maybe go to the Super Bowl against Philadelphia in New Orleans!

Sipe, being the competitor he is, sees a flash of Newsome in the middle. I know he's going for Newsome and not Logan. I stop breathing. I scream, clenching my fists, "Logan, Logan!" He doesn't hear me. He doesn't see Logan. My joy turns to vinegar in my mouth. Brian throws a wobbly pass. Mike Davis, their strong safety, is covering Ozzie man-to-man. Mike jumps in front of Ozzie and intercepts the pass in the end zone and, along with it, all our hopes and dreams. The people in the stands—70,000 of them—are shocked out of their ice cubes. I've never seen something die so fast. I can't even see good. All I can see is the interception, like a missile being picked off in midair before it can hit its target. Then my eyes focus on Sipe walking off the field with his head down and his helmet in his hands. It's like a silent, stop-action movie. Even though the crowd is screaming, I'm in my own silent world of private shock for a few seconds. I'm stunned. Sipe is totally bewildered. I put my arms around Brian and say, "Brian, I love you. You had a great year. I know how tough this is for you, but you gotta put it behind you." Brian looks at me like I'm crazy. In a few more seconds the game is over.

Now I've got that toughest of all coach's walks, the 40-yard walk off the field, through the tunnel, and into the locker room. The media would swarm all over me, all wanting to know why we threw the ball instead of kicking a field goal. As I walked through the tunnel, I began to pray. "Lord, I know You didn't call the pass play. I did. You didn't make the interception. They did. Please just give me wisdom now. I'm gonna get eaten alive in a few seconds."

When I faced the reporters, about one hundred in all, I didn't say much. I did what I had always instructed my team and my quarterback to do in interviews. I didn't get involved in the reasons for the decision. There's no way the media and the fans can identify with all the strategy in a game, particularly with the pressure during those decisions. Unless they have coached they really can't know how it is. The only thing that matters is if your strategy works. If it does, they call you a brilliant coach. If it doesn't, they second-guess you all the way into Lake Erie. A coach simply can't win against second-guessers. I guarantee you that if we had tried the field goal and missed, they would have said, "Hey, you've been winning with the pass all season. Brian already threw thirty touchdown passes during the season, and he eclipsed every Cleveland Browns passing record. Your mother told you a long time ago that the girl you take to the dance is the one you take home. Why didn't you stick to what was working for you and throw a pass?" I guarantee you, that would have been the reaction. If the pass had been completed for a touchdown, they would already have started constructing my statue at Public Square in downtown Cleveland.

I wanted to tell the media all the strategy, but it wouldn't have helped. I wanted to protect Brian during the press conference. We lost. That's all that mattered. There was nothing wrong with the call. The problem was the interception! Brian never should have thrown the ball in the middle of the field. He should have done exactly what he was told. The play was designed to go to Dave Logan. He couldn't have been any more open. End of story.

But Brian Sipe didn't play it that way to the media people. He talked a lot, probably too much. I had protected Brian in my comments, but he didn't return the favor. Later that year at the Senior Bowl, Don Shula told me he had been very upset with Brian's comments after our Raiders game. But I understand how it is when we get under pressure. We usually try to protect ourselves. Brian had never done anything like that before, and I just shrugged it off as a mistake in his judgment. We all make mistakes, as they say.

I waited a month to talk with Brian about it. He went to play and I went to coach in the Pro Bowl in Hawaii that year, and we had a long talk about it there. Brian admitted that he was under pressure and he shouldn't have spoken as he did to the press. He agreed 100 percent with the strategy of the Raiders game. But it was another of life's lessons for both of us. Brian is one of the greatest, most competitive athletes I ever coached.

The press conference was tough, no question about it. But even though Art Modell and Peter Hadhazy were happy to have been where they were, we all felt sad about being so close but not going all the way. The season was history.

In February, one of the Cleveland TV anchormen invited me to appear live on the six o'clock news. I got there early, and he took me to the cafeteria for a cup of coffee. He said, "Our station manager says that Cleveland has a real love affair with the Browns and Sam Rutigliano. Let's do something negative to zing Sam. It'll make good copy." He leveled with me because he wouldn't carry out his "zinging" orders.

I couldn't believe my ears. It surely gave me a good indication of how shallow people can be. By everybody's standards, we were winners. But we hadn't won it all. We were fair game. I felt that the football team belonged to the town. The radio and TV stations also belonged to the town. Why, in a moment of great joy and success, would they want to turn on us? It was too perplexing for me to fathom. Why wouldn't they want to push all the positive buttons on the wall rather than look for the negative ones? It was and still is a puzzlement to me. But it was a great lesson, too. In life, there are things that transcend football. There really is life after football. Life is always full of surprises.

Brian was eventually wooed away to the United States Football League in 1983. We had just beaten the San Diego Chargers in overtime. We were 3–1 for the year. That week we found out that Brian had flown to New York on his day off to talk about a move to the New Jersey Generals of the USFL. I read about it in the newspaper. Art Modell was furious. Of all the ill-timed things to happen. Never should something like that happen in the middle of a season.

Brian later came to my office and talked about it. He said, "Coach, this isn't going to affect the rest of my play for the Browns this season. It won't affect the way I prepare for a game or the way I play on Sunday."

I said, "Brian, I believe you. I know what kind of guy you are, but there are 48 other football players down in that locker room who are gonna think differently. Twenty-four are gonna be with you and twenty-four against you. Think about the can of worms you've opened up for the press. This will be better than the best soap opera on TV. This kind of situation should be dealt with prior to the start of the season. It's too tough to deal with during the season. It gets everybody distracted. We need all the concentration we can muster during the season. This will just drive a wedge into the center of what we're trying to do. Right now, we're 3–1 and in good position to get to the playoffs."

In all fairness to Brian, football has become a business, and he was starting on the down side of his career. His agent was simply trying to get him the best deal he could. That's his job. The USFL came along just at the right time for Brian. He wanted to know what the Browns would do for him during the next three or four years if he stayed, and that future prospect was too uncertain for him. The USFL guaranteed him a $2 million, three-year contract. He would have been stupid not to take it. But it made it tough for the Browns.

I was right about the soap opera. It brought chaos to the team. Is Brian going to sign, or isn't he? Is Paul McDonald going to replace him? It was "who's on first" time. The media had something to chew on. I mean, what the heck, they have to make a living, too. The soap opera played on and on for the entire year. The media people have a job, and that's to report the news. However, we don't have to feed them. Paul Brown said it best, "When you win, say nothing. When you lose, say less."

Most people don't know that Brian really wanted to stay with the Browns. But Art Modell wasn't about to guarantee Brian a $2 million contract. In retrospect, I really believe that Brian would have stayed with us if Art had made some kind of reasonable counteroffer. I believe he would have finished his distinguished career at Cleveland.

As I look back, with my 20/20 hindsight, I should have stood up on my hind legs and insisted that Art pay Brian long enough to train Paul McDonald. Then, if Paul could prove he was good enough to be the number-one quarterback for the Browns, it would have been worth it to Art Modell to pay Brian enough to keep him. I really believed that Paul was going to make it. But if Paul didn't work out, as eventually happened, Brian could have continued to win for us for several more years. So there's another mistake I made in not fighting to keep Brian with the Browns. He would have bridged the gap in '84, '85, and '86 in probably the poorest division in the NFL.

Knowing they wouldn't pay Brian enough, I went along with management and they went along with me because I felt we could win with McDonald. Each of us wanted to believe the other for our own reasons. If we had been able to keep Brian, we would have bridged the gap beautifully into the Bernie Kozar era. We were already on our way. Our defense was outstanding. We had built carefully. We had brought in Reggie Camp, Bob Golic, Carl Hairston, Clay Matthews, Chip Banks,

Eddie Johnson, Frank Minnifield, Hanford Dixon, and Chris Rockins. I knew we were going to have a great defense. I made a mistake in letting Brian get away. He would have been the insurance policy to help mold either Paul or Bernie into a winner, but we no longer had our insurance policy. The New Jersey Generals had Sipe, and we had McDonald.

In 1984, Paul's interceptions killed us. Many other things happened, but those interceptions! If you want to know how it feels to die on the sideline, try being a coach as he sees his quarterback throw an interception. You have to react, sometimes explode. It's unacceptable to a coach. It loses football games, it gives coaches ulcers, it gives owners heart attacks, it makes fans moan. Except for the interceptions that year, we would have been 6-2 or 5-3 at the worst in the middle of the season.

I could have had enough influence on Art Modell to keep Sipe. I'm sure Art wouldn't have paid him $2 million, but I believe I could have kept Brian. I believe Brian left because he felt I really didn't want him. It was another one of my mistakes. The absence of Brian Sipe hurt us more than anything else in 1984. You just can't win in the NFL if you don't have a great quarterback. In '78, '79, and '80, we were an average football team—or maybe slightly below average—but we had a great quarterback. In 1980 our defense was ranked twenty-sixth, but we won the division! Marty Schottenheimer was the defensive coach that year. Our defensive statistics were terrible. Yet, in 1984, we were ranked number one in defense. What was the difference? Marty would be the first to tell you the difference was the great defensive players we had in 1984. You never see a jockey carry a horse across the finish line. You gotta have players.

# CHAPTER TWENTY-ONE

# THE GIMME GENERATION

**Y**ou can't afford too many losing streaks. After the 1981 season with a 5–11 record, we wanted to make sure we came back strong. We opened the season in Seattle with a near-perfect game. Then, back in Cleveland against the Philadelphia Eagles, we lost in the final seconds. So, we were 1–1.

On the Monday following the Philadelphia game, all the coaches gathered at 8:00 AM. for the first meeting of the week. We huddled until one o'clock watching films and getting ready for our next game. Then there was a press conference at two o'clock when the players were due to report for a workout. I noticed that the players were there, talking in bunches but not making any attempt to get ready for a workout. The next thing I knew, all the players announced they were on strike and walked out of the locker room. Maybe I was naive and should have known they would strike, but I simply had no idea they would actually do it. They informed us they were not going to practice that day or any day until further notice, and they were not going to play the next game or any other game until further notice. They were, they said, on strike. They stayed out eleven weeks.

The players on each team were organized all over the United States. They wanted a new contract that would include 55 percent of the total revenue. Doug Dieken was the player representative for the Browns and Henry Shepherd was his assistant. Doug and Henry, along with Brian Sipe and several other veteran players, came to my office to assure me that they were going to stay together and stay in shape. I knew they were being unrealistic about the whole thing because many of the lower-paid players couldn't go very long without income during a strike. I had been through it before at New York. I knew there would be a split between the players if the strike dragged out too long. The economic pressure would get to the lower-paid ones.

The owners said it was preposterous for the players to ask for 55 percent of the revenue. They weren't in a mood to give away the store. The owners felt it was unfair because they had taken most of the financial risk right from the beginning. They said there was no way that the tail was going to wag the dog. As it turned out, the players settled for a lot less, and the Cleveland Browns lost millions of dollars in the process. Nobody won. The only thing that eventually helped the players was when the United States Football League started the following year. Then the NFL players' salaries went from an average of about $55,000 to about $241,000 today.

The other big problem in my life during the strike surfaced when we noticed that something ominous was happening to our youngest daughter, Kerry. She became increasingly rebellious at home, began failing in school, and didn't want to stay around home. It just wasn't like her. Finally we took her to the Cleveland Clinic where she was diagnosed as a bulimic, one who suffers from an eating disorder. That was before much was known about bulimia. Many young girls perceive themselves to be fat and unattractive, yet they seem to have insatiable appetites. So they gorge themselves with food and then induce vomiting, believing that this will cause them to lose weight. About 15 percent of them eventually commit suicide. We took the advice of the clinic's doctors and hospitalized Kerry for six months. The first three months of Kerry's hospitalization were during the players' strike, which gave me time to be with her at the clinic. Cynics might say there was no connection, but I have always been grateful to God that the strike gave me time to be with her. I'm not sure Barb would have been able to handle the crisis that was to come if I had been on my regular schedule.

Kerry was hospitalized before I went to training camp in July. On Tuesday night, prior to the Philadelphia game that year, we were to work late putting the game plan together. I almost never got home before 1:00 AM. on those kinds of nights. Before Kerry got sick I usually stayed at a hotel in Berea near the training camp because of the late hour. That night I got a terrifying call from Barb. She was incoherent.

"Sam, I, Kerry——"

"What is it, Barb? What's the matter?"

"It's Kerry, the hospital——"

"Barb, Barb, pull yourself together. Tell me what's the matter!"

"She tried to, oh, Sam, I——"

"For heaven's sake, Barb, tell me!"

"Kerry tried to commit suicide!"

My knees buckled beneath me. I felt sick. I couldn't find my voice for a second. "Barb, is she——"

"She's——they said she tried to——she cut her wrists!"

"Is she——?"

"She's all right, but——Kerry——oh, Sam, what are we going to do?"

After I hung up the telephone, I went into the training camp bathroom and locked myself in. In a few minutes I had to go into the room next door and be with my coaching staff for a meeting. They were all waiting for me. I got down on my knees and started to pray. "Lord, You've got to help us. Help Kerry. Help Barb and help me. How can we be going through something like this again? Nancy's death was bad enough, Lord. You know how long it took for us to recover from that. Help us, Lord." Soon I was crying. All I wanted to do was open the door, run out, get in my car, and drive to the hospital. I wanted to forget that I was a coach. My daughter needed me. When I recovered my composure, I called the hospital and got the story from a doctor.

God helped me through that evening. The next day Barb and I went to the hospital, and I winced at the sight of my sixteen-year-old daughter lying in a bed right beside the nurses' station where she could be watched. When Kerry saw Barb and me, she screamed, "I hate you for putting me here! I'm never going to get any better in here. I'm not ever going back to school either!"

Seeing her like that tore my heart out. Football seemed so irrelevant at that moment. Everything seemed irrelevant. The only thing that mattered to me right then was for Kerry to be healed. After everybody calmed down and we talked further to the doctor, he said Kerry hadn't seriously harmed herself, but she was sending a clear message to us with her attempt. Kerry hadn't "slashed" her wrists so much as she had scratched them. But the doctor said we had to take her actions seriously because sometimes a young person like Kerry might intend only to send a message but could fatally hurt herself. Kerry was desperately trying to get our attention. Her strategy worked!

I was devastated. At that moment I wanted to throw in the towel. I didn't care if I ever coached again, and I had to go back the next day to coach the Browns into readiness for the Philadelphia game. I was looking at a season that had only fifteen games. God didn't cause the strike, but it certainly worked out that I had time to be with Kerry at a very critical time in her life. Bulimia is for real. Barb and I may not have been able to cope with the whole situation as well as we did if I had been gone my usual number of days. The demands on a coach during the season are enormous. Thank God Kerry has improved greatly and leads a full and exciting life now.

After the strike, we beat the New England Patriots in a very close game our first time out in Cleveland Municipal Stadium. Then we lost to San Diego and Dallas. I had to make a major decision about Brian Sipe, who wasn't playing well at all. Two years before that, he was voted the Most Valuable Player. Same guy, two years later, but not the same results.

I replaced Brian, a major competitor in the NFL, with Paul Mcdonald, a young, unproven quarterback. Fortunately, Paul won two games in a row. We were 4–4, and I looked like a genius for a few hours. We beat Houston in Houston and qualified for the playoffs, even though it was a strike year. It looked like we had a chance.

Just when you think things have stabilized, something always seems to crash in on you. We decided to fly to Los Angeles to prepare for the Raiders game in Anaheim. We sure didn't want to stay in Cleveland that week in December when we could practice in the sunshine. We were about thirty minutes from Los Angeles, and I was daydreaming in my seat. I thought about the two huge crises I had survived that year and wondered what else could possibly go wrong. I got an immediate answer when I looked down the aisle of the plane and saw a person lying on the floor with people gathered around. I got up from my seat and said aloud, "Oh, no! It's Art Modell!" The doctors were hovering over him, and it looked like he had had a heart attack.

An ambulance met us at the airport and took Art and me to the hospital. I stayed with him that night until we learned that he was out of danger for the time being. It was a warning to Art. The doctors advised him to have a heart catheterization, but he put it off. Eventually he did have a heart attack but, thank God, he made it. That was a difficult year all the way around. But even with all those crises, there would be more.

# CHAPTER TWENTY-TWO

# COMMUNICATION IS NONVERBAL

**A** professional football coach never knows where he's going to be from year to year. As you climb the ladder looking for that head coaching position, you have to be open for opportunities. Then when you finally get your dream job, you have to keep looking over your shoulder because they're coming after you in bunches. Don't ever look behind you. Someone is always following. Owners and management are constantly trying to reinvent the wheel.

Four coaches left our staff after the 1982 season. Len Fontes, the defensive secondary coach, went to the New York Giants. Paul Hackett, our quarterback coach, went to the San Francisco 49ers. Rich Kotite, our receiver coach, went to the New York Jets. Rod Humenuik went to the Kansas City Chiefs. Today Paul Hackett is the offensive coordinator for the Dallas Cowboys. Rod Humenuik is assistant head coach and offensive coordinator for the New England Patriots. Rich Kotite is the offensive coordinator for the New York Jets. Len Fontes is the defensive secondary coach and is also in charge of pass defense for the New York Giants.

Since we lost some very fine men, we had to build a new staff almost from scratch. We picked up Larry Weaver, the offensive coordinator for the San Diego Chargers, who proved to be a big plus for our football team. They say you can't tell the players without a program. There ought to be a special program about the coaches!

We started the 1983 season with a lot of hope but with a lot of controversy regarding our quarterback situation. The media people wanted to know who was going to be our starting quarterback. Brian Sipe was our starter for the first game at Cleveland against the Minnesota Vikings. It was obvious during the preseason that Brian was a great competitor and the players had confidence in him. As soon as I made the decision to start Brian, I called Paul to my office and privately told him. I also told him I believed he, Paul, was our quarterback of the future.

I was very much aware of the prowling scouts of the United States Football League who were looking for players, especially quarterbacks. The irony for me, as I later learned, was that Donald Trump wanted Brian to be the quarterback for the New Jersey Generals. Along with that development, Paul McDonald's agent, Lee Steinberg, was already moving in for a deal for Paul. So, not only were we in the midst of a quarterback controversy, but we could possibly lose both our quarterbacks. We knew Brian was being wooed heavily. If we didn't match his USFL offer, we would lose him. Paul felt that if Brian was going to stay with the Browns, he was going to fly the coop himself. Paul had already played three years behind Brian, and he was anxious to get on with his career as a starting quarterback.

We lost the Vikings game 27–21. In the fourth quarter we had the ball on their 15-yard line with less than a minute to go. The stage was set. It was the guys in the white hats all over again. It was Brian Sipe at his best. I felt that all we had to do was throw one ball in the end zone for a touchdown and it would be all over. Brian had done it so many times before. It should have been a piece of cake for him. But Brian got a little bit out of sync and tried to force the ball. He threw an interception, and we lost the game.

In the locker room after the game I broke one of my own rules. I always tried to keep my mouth shut if I was angry. I always tried to wait until I cooled down before I spoke. I always stressed the importance of saying positive things. But I was absolutely livid. I yelled to the players, "We should have won this game! There's no way we should have lost. I'm the guy with all the pressure. I have to answer to the media, I have to answer to the owners, I have to answer to you guys, I have to answer to the whole world! I'm the guy who wears the sombrero! I'm the guy who takes all the heat!" I was living proof of the statement that "we're all horses' tails at least five minutes a day, but the secret is not to exceed the limit." That day in the locker room I exceeded the limit.

I thought about it all Sunday evening. When I went to the team meeting Monday morning, I went after them again. I was mad. I repeated my remarks about being the guy who wears the sombrero and who takes all the heat. I thought about it all day Tuesday, which was the players' day off. I began to regret my negative outburst to the guys. I couldn't wait for Wednesday to arrive so I could tell the players I was sorry and I had made a mistake in chewing them out the way I did.

Our team meeting that Wednesday was to start at 10:05. I had my agenda all set. I would start off with my apology and then review our goals for the week and the next game. That meeting was to be very important. It would set the tone for the rest of the week. I was anxious to see the guys since I had settled down and accepted our loss that past Sunday.

I opened the door of the meeting room and got shocked out of my sneakers. There were all forty-nine football players grinning at me, all wearing sombreros! What could I do? I broke up. Everybody broke up. It was a great lesson for me. At least 75 percent of all communication is nonverbal. The guys were saying to me, "Hey, Coach, we win together, and we lose together. You ain't the only guy on the sideline who has something to lose." I thanked them for bringing me back to where I needed to be.

That season had great thrills of victory and bruising agonies of defeat. I benched Sipe and brought in McDonald, but he didn't do the job. There was always the threat of Sipe leaving at any time. His agent's open negotiations with Don Trump caused near chaos within our organization. A player absolutely must have his contract settled in the off-season. There's no way he can concentrate while he's playing for one team if he's considering joining another one. We needed to be fully involved in winning our football games, but we were distracted every day. We weren't all pulling together toward the same flag. Paul McDonald was singing that old familiar song, "Play me or trade me." Football wasn't as much fun as it used to be.

In the middle of the season we were 5-5, and the wolves were howling. The fans were beginning to go after me personally. But Brian got hot, and the defense got hot enough to win three in a row. We were 8-5 with a very good chance to get into the playoffs. Next was Denver, but we had never beaten them there. All we had to do was beat Denver and we were in the playoffs. We lost.

The following week we went to Houston, a team not doing much that year. Mike Pruitt hadn't fumbled once that year to date. He caught an almost terminal case of fumblitis during the Houston game. He fumbled five, count 'em, five times! We're down 24-6. We come back and go ahead 27-24! It's in the bag after such a comeback, right? Wrong! We could have iced the chance to make the playoffs. We lost. That made us 8-7.

So what does that leave for the last game of the year? Pittsburgh! At least we're playing them at Cleveland. We *have* to win this game. Brian has a very good game, and we win it.

Now we're 9–7. About five teams in the league are 9–7. We're still alive. If New England, scheduled to play right after our game that day, can beat Seattle in Seattle, we go to the playoffs. Seattle beat New England. Out of four or five teams that were 9–7 in the NFL, we were the only team that didn't make the playoffs.

The quarterback rodeo finally played itself out that year when I had talks with both Brian Sipe and Paul McDonald. When Paul came to my office, I told him, "Paul, your handshake is your character. Your word is your character. I want you to know right now that, even if Brian leaves, if you don't live up to the agreement in that contract, I don't care if you stay here or not because we're not moving one inch off dead center." Paul showed me a lot of character and a lot of class when he signed his contract.

Right after the Pittsburgh game, Brian came to my office and said, "Coach, I want to be the first to tell you that I've signed with the New Jersey Generals. I don't want you to read about it in the papers first. I couldn't turn it down. They gave me a three-year contract with a $2 million guarantee." What do you say to a guy who stands in front of you with a message like that? Here's a guy who was going to make more money in three years than most people will see in a lifetime. Am I going to tell him I think he's making a mistake? I told him I couldn't blame him. But I shoulda tried to keep Brian Sipe. Coulda, woulda, shoulda.

Our division was not the same as it had been from 1978 through 1981. All the teams were struggling. Bradshaw was gone from the Steelers, Kenny Anderson wasn't playing the way he had in the past, and Ken Stabler was gone. Brian Sipe could have kept us winning, even if he was a "descending" player. Records of 8–8 and 9–7 now would win the division championship. Coulda, woulda. I shoulda kept Sipe. He coulda helped groom McDonald, we coulda won the division, I woulda still been the coach of the Cleveland Browns. Coulda, woulda, shoulda.

The year 1983 was really something overall. Art Modell had a heart attack that year. I stayed with him during his surgery, which went well. When we saw that he was out of danger, Barb and I started out driving to our vacation home in Charleston, South Carolina, for a rest. We got as far as Charlotte, North Carolina, where I called back to Cleveland to see how Art was doing. When I learned that he had taken a turn for the worse, I flew back to Cleveland to be with him while Barb drove on to Charleston with our daughters.

Art had had some postoperative complications so I spent the entire week with him. He wasn't able to ventilate. I sat with some of the finest pulmonary anesthesiologists in the world, listening with great interest. Pat Modell and John, their son, also were in the meeting. I felt very sorry for Pat. I prayed a lot that week. I was with Pat and John every day. There were times when we didn't know for sure if Art would make it.

Toward the end of that week, I was sitting in the waiting room with Pat while John was praying in the chapel. The doctor came to tell Pat that, although Art's condition was not the best, it looked like he would make it after all. It was a very emotional moment for us. Art was going to make it. Pat looked at me and said, "Thank God."

I felt a strong kinship with Pat at that moment and thought back to when our little Nancy was killed. I knew the anguish Pat had experienced and was so happy for her when she received the encouraging news. My silent prayer at the time was that she and Art would find the peace that God had given Barb and me after our own tragedy.

The year 1983 was not routine.

# CHAPTER TWENTY-THREE

# ONE FOOT IN THE GRAVE, ONE ON A BANANA PEEL

**S**pringtime is supposed to bring new beginnings, new life, and good news, but those good things don't always follow. As soon as Rich Kotite, our receiver coach, came into my office one day in the spring of 1982, I felt my stomach rumble. My office was always open to the staff and the players. But Rich closed the door behind him and locked it. He had my full attention. Rich was a close friend with whom I had worked at the New Orleans Saints. (He's now the offensive coordinator for the New York Jets.) He's from Brooklyn, and of course, we communicated easily. Growing up in Brooklyn teaches you to communicate with people in order to survive. Rich was as perceptive as any coach on the staff. When he came to see me, which wasn't often, he always had something important to say.

When he closed and locked the door, I immediately thought some other team had made him an offer. Or perhaps he had a serious health problem again. After all, he did have a brain tumor in 1981. I took Rich very seriously all the time because he was a straight shooter and reliable.

When he sat down, he said, "Coach, we have a big problem."

"What kind of problem, Rich?"

"I don't know where to start."

"Start from the beginning. My mind is jumping in ten directions at once. The last time we had a conversation like this you had a brain tumor. Are you OK?"

"Yes, I'm fine. It's not about me or my family. It's about our football team."

"Give it to me, Rich."

"Sam, we've got a drug problem."

I looked at Rich and said, "You gotta be kidding. Whattaya mean, drug problem? I'm sure there might be some people we could help because they might be recreational users or some who are experimenting with marijuana." I heard myself issuing the classic response of denial like any father who first hears the dreaded news about his children's drug involvement.

"No, Sam. We've got people into drugs on this team in a big way."

"Now wait, Rich, that's a heck of a statement for you to make. Does anyone else know about this?"

"No, not on the staff. Some players came to me and said there are users on the team. They wouldn't tell me who the players are, but they're here. I have my own thoughts about it, but I think you should know first."

I thought back to Carl Eller's visit and warning. My thoughts started really spinning. Maybe this was the beginning of some kind of an answer as to why we lost eleven games last year. "Rich, this is going to require a lot of thought. I appreciate your telling me. Information is like eggs—the fresher the better. Please assure me that you won't say anything to anyone else until we can think it through." When Rich left, I knew I had to talk to Art Modell. Within a few hours I had called Art and set up an appointment at his stadium office.

I walked into the big downtown office that overlooked Lake Erie and found Art waiting and curious. After all, I had driven all the way from my Baldwin-Wallace campus office on the West Side of Cleveland.

After we said hello, I said, "Art, I've just learned on good authority that we have some suspected drug users on our team."

"Who's involved? How bad is it?"

"I don't know the names yet, but I've seen the tip of what may be an iceberg."

"What do you think we should do?"

"There are two perspectives we can have. First, as human beings in leadership positions, we have a responsibility to help these guys. Second, from an economic perspective, when players get suspended for drug use, how do you replace them? The NFL suspended the Bengals' Ross Browner, their defensive end, and Pete Johnson, their fullback, for a month. How do you replace superstars? You have to redraft and re-sign players. You have to repay big bonuses and salaries, and it all takes time and money. Just from an economic standpoint, Art, it's worth it to do whatever we can to combat this thing."

"You're right, Sam. What do you think we should do?"

"The league office has already asked each team to use local psychiatrists who have experience with chemical and alcohol dependency to act as consultants. I think we should set up a formal organization and get professional help to try to cure those who are ill and prevent the straight ones from becoming involved in drugs."

"If you think it's that bad."

"I do, Art."

"Then your idea sounds like a good one."

Art couldn't have been more helpful. From the start, he was very cooperative, and the Inner Circle was born.

It didn't take us long to have a fantastic organizational chart starting with Art Modell as the chairman of the board. Next, I was the CEO. Dr. Greg Collins was the expert in the field of alcohol and chemical dependency. Calvin Hill, Paul Warfield, and Ted Chappelle were involved in the employee assistance program. Tom Petersberg was the spiritual leader.

Our thoughts were that the players could be rehabilitated—physically, emotionally, mentally, socially, and spiritually—through education. The Inner Circle was basically a support group that utilized the dynamics of peer pressure as well as counseling and education. Players with serious drug or alcohol addiction would be required to undergo treatment at detoxification centers. When a player began the aftercare program, he was required to attend three meetings each week.

We had something in place, but how were we going to get the users to step forward and reveal their problems? Most pro athletes are like caterpillars. They follow the leader. Peer approval is more important than self-approval. We go with the tide most of the time. I once read of an experiment in which a row of caterpillars were placed head to tail on the rim of a big flowerpot. They followed each other around the rim for seven days and seven nights. Ample food and water were just inside the rim of the flowerpot. We follow the followers. We sometimes behave the same way as the caterpillars. Habits, patterns, and ways of thinking are easy to follow when "everybody's doing it." We need to step out of line at times and look ahead to see who we are following. In the case of the caterpillars, they all died, circling food and water.

A football team is made of three circles: (1) 80 percent are in the middle in a big circle, and they usually go with the flow; (2) 10 percent are negative; and (3) 10 percent are positive. The negative ones always see a bottle as half empty. No matter how much you preach to them or how well you treat them, they always want more. If you give them an inch, they want a yard. If you give them a wrist, they want your entire arm. They'll go right up to your armpit if you let them. Then there's always that other 10 percent who are leaders. They're always pushing the positive buttons. To them, the bottle is always half full. The secret of good relationships between coaches and players is to get the majority of players to swing along with the 10 percent who are always positive. Once you get your football team moving in the direction toward that attitude, the 10 percent who are negative discover that most of the players don't want to hear their negative statements in the locker room. Their influence dies.

I started finding out more and more about this big puzzle, putting one little piece after another together. Every day I talked to the equipment man and the trainer. They kept their eyes and ears open for me.

We began to improve in monitoring our players. During the season, a professional football player has to keep a very rigorous, demanding, and disciplined schedule. It was easy to measure a consistent performance that the drug user replaces with inconsistency. Players who once strove to be the best were satisfied with much less. We noticed tremendous mood swings in a player who previously displayed a stable personality.

It was important for each assistant coach to monitor his own groups. On out-of-town trips the coaches handled bed checks of their own groups rather than have one or two coaches do them all. That way coaches could sit down and visit with their players. Assistant coaches spend a lot of time with their groups all week long. They could watch for anything unusual, such as reporting to practice late, arriving late at airports, sleeping in meetings, not participating in meetings, and not measuring up to par in daily practice as the coaches evaluated them each day on film. It's hard for a user to escape in that kind of environment. The problem is that most teams do not train their coaches, trainers, equipment men, and everyone else in the organization to detect the telltale signs of drug or alcohol abuse. If they did, the early warning signs would expedite the need for help.

I can remember arguing with the other coaches in our NFL meetings in Hawaii. They would say, "After the game, the players want to relax and be refreshed. So we'll stand at the entrance to the plane and hand out only two beers to each player."

I said, "Is that what they pay you hundreds of thousands of dollars for, to hand out cans of beer? Here we are talking about alcohol abuse, which is a bigger problem than drug abuse, and we're condoning and even paying for the beer? You crazy? Sure, players will come to you and ask why they can't have beer on the plane. They'll say they can go out and buy it after the plane lands. I'll tell you what I'm gonna tell them. I'll tell them, sure, they can go out and buy it, but I'll never be involved in a drug-and-alcohol prevention program with one hand and give my players beer with the other. That's stupid!" All of us on the Browns staff, including Art Modell, agreed that we shouldn't have alcohol on the planes.

All these were the beginnings of positive steps. We began to be very careful about who was included on the crews of the chartered air flights. We wanted to make sure they wouldn't enable the players to drink or use drugs while on the flights. I found out that one player walked on the plane carrying a bottle of pop with a lot of gin in it. One of the flight attendants helped that player conceal his booze.

Not until we began watching the players more closely did they realize we cared enough about their welfare to take some positive steps. Sure, some of the players bellyached about being treated like kids, but they were in the minority. Our approach to the problem also reassured the positive guys that the rules can't be broken. It's always disheartening to them to see guys breaking rules and coaches looking the other way. Before this, we were like parents who said, "Look, I know you have a problem with drugs at the high school, but it's not a problem with *my* kid." Or "Thank God my son was simply drunk at the emergency room the other night and it was just marijuana." Or "It couldn't be my daughter you saw in the gynecologist's office. My daughter's not pregnant." Blindman's bluff. We didn't want to hear it. We didn't believe it when we did hear it. It's something you just wish would go away. They call it an illusion of immunity. But finally we stopped acting like ostriches and took our heads out of the sand.

Ted Chappelle was an important part of this. He established a system of security with people reporting to him. His philosophy was that surveillance was important and it would deter players. Some of the players would tell him about seeing known drug dealers watching the team practice. During Saturday practices at the stadium, the players often brought their families to watch. It was family day, a leisurely, fun time for the players' wives and children, parents, and relatives. They brought them into the locker room and gave them autographs.

All the while, just outside the stadium, the drug dealers hung around like a bunch of wild jackals waiting to creep in. They followed the players all over the USA, taking other flights and following the team to the same cities. Professional athletes comprise a big, important market for the pushers. First of all, the players have plenty of cash. Second, the dealers like to be associated with professional athletes. Besides, the players bring additional customers to the dealers and receive "discounts" when they buy their own drugs. The dealers get an ever-widening stranglehold on the players.

Although Ted Chappelle wasn't hired to be a detective, he gave us a lot of professional advice on how to proceed. He showed us the right process to follow as we considered players in the draft. We wanted to know *before* the draft whether the player ever had a drug problem. The NFL teams had already made a lot of mistakes in this regard. You have to draft quality people to build your football team. Ted's advice was a tremendous educational experience. Once your eyes are opened to some of the patterns to watch for, it's like seeing with corrective glasses the first time. Some things you never saw before become very plain.

So, what began with a conversation with Rich Kotite, in which I tended to shrug off the possibility of users on our team, grew into a major project. Before my eyes were opened to the magnitude of the problem, I tended to think it was just a stage young guys went through experimenting with a little pot here, a little beer there. Little did I know. One thing I did know: we needed to pay attention to the problem because it did exist and it wasn't going away.

The next step was education; everybody agreed on that. We brought Carl Eller in for a series of lectures for our players. We got reams of written material showing the evils of drugs and alcohol. During our three-day minicamps in the off-season, we hit the subject hard. But with all our efforts, I finally realized that a drug user is going to stay in the closet, concealed. Sure, he'll listen to all the lectures and come to all the meetings, but he won't step forward until he has a close brush with death or some other scary thing in his life that was drug-induced.

Carl kept telling me, "Coach, in the thirteen years I played in the NFL I used every kind of drink and drug you can name, and I still played. I used alcohol, marijuana, cocaine, uppers, downers, you name it. Hey, as long as I could play good, nobody cared. What bugs me now is how much better I might have been had I stayed clean. The thing I feared the most was retribution. If they found out I was a user, they would have kicked me off the team. That would have killed me. But there was no one I could go to. I couldn't trust anyone. I had to keep it to myself."

What Carl feared the most had been very real in the sports world up to that time. Players who had drug or alcohol problems were simply fired in the 1950s and 1960s. There was no sentiment of understanding or compassion toward them. Even when Paul Horning and Alex Karras were caught gambling, they were suspended for a year. No wrist slapping in those days. Everybody thought that spots on the leopard never changed, so you might as well get rid of them as soon as you know they're problem drinkers or drug users. That was the prevailing attitude among owners and coaches in those days. Nobody felt those problems were diseases. There are people today who will say that cocaine use is not a disease. *Webster's Dictionary* says a *disease* is "a particular destructive process in the body, with a specific cause and characteristic symptoms." Drug use is a disease.

Suppose you have congestion in your chest and you go to a doctor about it. He examines you and says, "You're smoking too many cigarettes. You'd better stop, or you'll get cancer of the lungs. All cancer is bad, but cancer of the lungs is the worst." So, you don't listen to the doctor, and in five years you've got cancer of the lungs. You go back to the doctor and say, "Doc, you've got to treat me; you've got to cure me!"

The same thing is true with marijuana and cocaine users. These people are sick. They have "a particular destructive process in the body." Sure, it's self-imposed, but it's still a disease. The problem with alcohol and drug users is that they don't think they're sick so they're not going to come forward. I saw then that it was going to take a lot of education. I hoped that at least one person would eventually come forward. I knew that we had to be part of the solution or we would be part of the problem.

I recognized that we were doing about as much as we possibly could, but I still felt helpless because I wanted to do much more. It was like watching someone drowning and knowing that all I could do was let the water out of the pool. I couldn't just jump in and react immediately. It was premature. We were still in the dark. We knew we had users on the team, but we didn't know which ones.

I knew that if we tried too much police work, we would simply drive the users deeper into the closet. I had heard that some coaches used German Shepherds to sniff around in the locker rooms. Too often coaches begin to moralize to the users. "How could you do this to yourself? Don't you know you'll ruin your career? There are hundreds of players who want to take your place. Less than 1 percent of all the players in America who stay in high school and college make it into the NFL. Do you realize just how great an opportunity you have? Think of the kind of money you can earn the rest of your career. Most of you come from the lower socioeconomic sector of America, and now you're moving into the upper 2 percent of all wage earners. If you take care of yourself, you can play for ten years. You'll be set for life, for cryin' out loud!'' When a coach tells a user something like that, the player can't wait to get out of the office to get another snort of cocaine or another joint of marijuana to allay his guilt.

The other thing a coach can't do is diagnose drug users. Coaches aren't qualified to do that. I guarded against this temptation myself. I made sure the people who dealt with the players every day, such as the assistant coaches, equipment men, and trainers, simply monitored the players and kept track of unusual behavior over a period of time. Sooner or later a pattern would emerge that I could track.

Then we got our first break. One day a player walked into my office and asked if he could talk to me. Players walk into the coach's office all the time, and they talk about a lot of things. Some want to know why they're sitting on the bench. They want to know what they have to do to improve their situation with the team. They talk about money, about getting a girl pregnant, about school and all kinds of private problems. I noticed immediately how nervous he was. He was perspiring as he said, "Coach, can I talk to you?"

"Sure, sit down."

He was vague. He stuttered as he tried to make small talk about his weight program and about how fine he was and how he hoped he would be able to contribute to the team this next year. It was obvious to me that he was leading up to something. I was waiting for the punch line, like "Hey, Coach, I need to borrow some money," or "I don't want to get involved in the off-season program because I want to go home," or "I can't make it to minicamp because of a personal problem," or "I've got some girl in a family way," or "I've got some kind of venereal disease." Mind you, this kind of thing didn't happen every day, but over a period of time these situations accumulate. Still I wanted to be careful and sensitive. *Who knows what he has on his mind?* I fought off impatience as he scooted around in his chair and seemed very ill at ease. I didn't want to be like one of the assistant coaches who came to me all excited one day and said, "Coach, there's a guy sleeping in the meeting. He's gotta be on cocaine." I didn't want to jump to conclusions and overreact. I knew it was important to have only one person confront the player. In my opinion, this is the job of the head coach.

He finally stopped squirming and looked me right in the eye, "Coach, I have a very serious problem. I don't know what to do about it."

"Whatever you want to tell me. Take your time."

"I don't know if I can trust you."

"Look, we're not gonna stay in here all day beating around the bush, and I'm not gonna preach to you."

"Well, I——man, it's hard to say——I mean——"

"Hey, all I can tell you is that you can trust me."

"Coach——" He looked away and remained silent.

"Listen, I'm not gonna say what your problem is. I *know* what the problem is. But what you need to do now is understand that I am not going to moralize to you. I am not going to diagnose. I am only going to say one thing to you. You *must* trust me. If you don't, your problem will eventually end your career and kill you. It's a dead end." I knew this man had reached the end of his rope and couldn't handle life by himself. Otherwise, he never would have stepped forward.

"Coach, it's so hard——" He looked away again.

"Just trust me, will you?"

He said, "Coach, I've got a drug problem."

I knew I was looking into the eyes of a drug addict. I knew that addicts denied their addiction. This man had reached the first important step of acknowledging his problem. I also knew that addicts were pathological liars. I knew I had to be careful. I said, "Look, two things you need to know. First, you can trust me. Second, you won't lose your job unless you refuse to help yourself. We'll help anyone who wants to help himself. I'll get you with complete anonymity to the doctor at the Cleveland Clinic. You won't tell the secretary your name. You'll just go to see him. He'll evaluate you. I want you to know this: once he evaluates you, you must do exactly what he says. I know it's too early for you to know you can trust me, but you really don't have any alternative, do you?"

"No, Coach."

I knew what was going on in his mind. He was afraid, afraid of what might happen to him. I remembered Carl Eller relating his fears of retribution. I didn't want to scare this man away. This was the opening we had been waiting for. I didn't want to probe too much now. I didn't want him to ask a lot of questions about what procedure he would have to follow. All I wanted him to do at that moment was agree to see the doctor. I said, "The doctor is a qualified expert. Let's get his opinion before we do anything else."

He looked at me again, "Coach, will I have to go off to some drug rehabilitation place or something? All the guys will notice if I'm gone for a while."

"Look, I don't know anything more right now than this: you have to see the doctor before anything else can happen. I'll tell you one thing, getting to the doctor is something you have to do. You have to make sure that you do what he says."

When he got up to leave, I walked around my desk and put my arm around him and said, "I love you. It took guts for you to come in here to see me. I really do want to help you."

I knew that his coming to see me was the most important thing to happen to date in our antidrug program. I knew that he would talk to other players as soon as he left my office. He would probably talk to his friends who were also using drugs. It was absolutely essential that he left my office believing he could trust me. He could tell the other users that the coach understood and was fair. He could tell them that he was given an opportunity to take a first step toward recovery and still carry on with his career.

I really didn't know how he felt or what he believed. It was my first confrontation with a player who had a drug problem. I learned later that it was important to keep such a conversation short. The poor guy left my office in a pool of sweat. He was really scared. Can you imagine what it took for him to come forward? He could have lost it all. He was alone. He was sick and scared. I tried to comfort and assure him. It was like the attendant waiting to escort the convict on death row into the gas chamber. The attendant said, "Don't worry. It'll be all over quickly." And then the convict answered, "How do you know?"

The young man went to see the doctor who confirmed to me that he had a serious cocaine addiction. He immediately called Carl Eller in Minneapolis who arranged to admit the player to a rehab center. The next day the player was on a plane to a rehab center and was scheduled to be there for one month.

Each week I talked to the player on the telephone. The first week, he seemed very withdrawn and afraid. He didn't really want to talk to me. Then, week by week, he changed noticeably. By the third week, he was as excited as a little kid. It was miracle of healing. He was on a spiritual mountaintop. He cried; he cared; he thanked me for sending him there;

he thanked me for Carl Eller, and Art Modell. He couldn't wait to get back to Cleveland and influence other users to stop their suicidal lifestyles. He just knew he would be a much better football player. He had taken the first step on his journey of a thousand miles and was on his way.

We were very much aware of the dangers of his coming down off the mountaintop and going back into the real world. In the rehab center he was sheltered; drug pushers couldn't get to him. He would need to have local support. He was the first to step forward. He was very thankful to us, but I felt very grateful to him for starting the exodus out of the drug jungle, leading the way for the others who eventually came into the Inner Circle. He had been the forerunner, the market tester for all the other users. He was proof that the system worked and that users could step forward and keep their anonymity and their jobs.

Carl Eller constantly told the players that a successful alcohol and drug program depends on having a head coach you can trust and an owner who won't fire you. We had both. And we had prevention, intervention, and aftercare. When a former user comes out of the thirty days of rehab therapy, he is very vulnerable and had better be involved in aftercare. The temptations will be great. He will need all the help and support he can get. Not only will the pushers try to get back to him, but so will some of his friends who are still users. They want their friend to take up where he left off before he went to dry out. Maybe some of them want him to resume buying from their pusher because they get a discount on their own drugs. Sometimes it works like a pyramid club or chain letter. The more people you can introduce to the pusher, the greater will be the discount on your own drug needs. It's vicious. The recovering drug addict simply must be protected when he goes back into the real world. He must totally avoid his previous environment.

With the young man sent off to the drug rehab center, I was left to wonder who, if anyone, would be next to step forward.

# CHAPTER TWENTY-FOUR

# CONFRONTATION

**D**uring the time one of our users was away at a drug rehab center, I talked with him on the telephone for a long time several days apart. After two weeks he was on a spiritual and mental high. He was beginning to be free of chemical dependency. He was beginning to see that he might make it after all. We both had high hopes. We had a great mutual trust going for us, which I assumed would open the way for him to call me at any time he was concerned about anything.

When my secretary announced that so-and-so was on the line, my heart jumped a few beats. Why would he be calling me when we had just talked not too long ago?

I said, "Hello."

He tried to talk but could only cry. He was desperate. I had been hoping against hope that he would hang in and make it. The sound of his voice brought chills to my spine. Had he strayed from the straight and narrow way? Had he left the rehab center? He could hardly speak to me. He was almost incoherent. I feared the worst.

"Coach, I know we have an agreement that we won't use anybody's name, but there's one player I'm really worried about. I think he's gonna go off the deep end. It may already be too late for him."

I said, "Look, this man's life is more important than our code or our agreement. Who is it?"

"I can't, I mean, Coach, I'm sorry. It's ———. He's in desperate trouble. He has lots of problems with his family, he has problems with drugs and drug dealers. He's got problems in every phase of his life. All his walls are cracking. He's in quicksand right now, and he doesn't know who to turn to. I've called him and talked with him and told him he can trust you. But he is worried that he can't trust anyone. He's worried that you'll get rid of him if he comes to you or that Art Modell will get rid of him if he finds out about the drug problem. He just doesn't trust the organization, and he's worried about getting fired."

I immediately remembered Carl Eller's fear of retribution and how he covered up his addiction for years because of it. I said, "The most important thing for you right now is to struggle with your own drug problem. You need to work on it one day at a time. I promise you that I'll think about what you've just told me and I'll take action, one way or the other."

I replaced the telephone and reflected on the past when we were preparing to play a very important game. Thinking back to this game, the importance of preparation stuck in my mind.

Every week, we introduce a new game plan to our players. We always wanted our players to absorb the game plan, to think about it, to visualize it, to keep it in mind day and night as we approached the game day. We always filmed the practice sessions so everybody could look at the film the next day. It's absolutely imperative for the players to concentrate on the game plan. If every businessman could have film of himself every day as he goes about his business, he would be much more efficient. We always said that "the big eye doesn't lie." When the players came in the day after practice for the meetings, I could point out mistakes to be corrected. No player could deny making a mistake that was clearly shown on the film.

While concentration is very important for the players, they also have to be enthusiastic. In fact, part of the game plan is to be enthusiastic. I wanted the players to be so interested in the game plan that they might make suggestions to change it. Many times the quarterback made such suggestions. When we saw the practice films, we could often see the wisdom of making some changes. After all, the quarterback knew more than we did sometimes because he was the guy who had to go out there and execute the plan.

The third important thing about the game plan is execution. If the players pay close attention to detail during the week's preparation and develop enthusiasm about the game plan, the only thing left is execution. The players made some of the best suggestions we ever had during the week of preparation and during the course of the game on Sunday. Knowing the game plan and helping "author" it with pride of authorship are crucial for a team.

I remembered that the coaches had said some players were sleeping in the meetings. Whenever you see a player dozing in an important meeting, you think back to the mistakes he made during practice. You think back to the examination he failed when a coach tested him. You think back to a time when a coach asked him a question in front of the entire squad and heard his incorrect answer. Everybody else on the squad knows the answer and there's a player who can't give the right answer.

Visualize a game. The quarterback drops back to pass. The five offensive linemen pick up the rushing linemen. The fullback picks up the raging bull of a linebacker ripping through in a nasty mood. The receivers get off the line of scrimmage and fight to get open. Downfield, the receiver is one-on-one with the corner. He has him beat. The quarterback reads the defense and spots the receiver breaking open. The protection is solid. We have the 2.8 seconds we need to complete the pass. Pass protection is the most important part of pass offense. You have to keep your quarterback on his feet and not on the ground. The defense not only want to sack your quarterback, they count the times they knock him down. That's what separates the great ones, the courage to stay in the pocket and concentrate downfield.

I yell, "He's open! He's open! Get the ball to him!" He sees him. The ball is up. Now I'm running along the sideline. "Catch it! Catch it! Catch it! Catch it!" What a fabulous sight. Touchdown. What an exhilarating feeling! Everything worked just as we planned it. That ought to shut those fans up. We showed 'em. "Nice catch! Perfect throw!" Wait a minute, wait a minute! What's that? "No, no! There's a flag, there's a flag! They musta been offside, right? What? What? Cleveland penalty? Oh, no! Who was it? Who was it? I'll kill 'im! Whose number? Oh, no!" That's what can happen if a player does not concentrate. He is not on the same page with the other ten guys on the field.

As I flashed back on these scenes I said to myself, *It's all beginning to fit together. It's like a Sherlock Holmes mystery. A clue here, another one there.* It was all right there in front of us, and we had been too blind to see it. But since we had been educated about chemical abuse, all the pieces started to fit.

So, when a player in rehab called me about another teammate, I had no concern whatsoever about the code. Who cared about the code? Who cared about whatever agreements we had? Who cared about what the other players thought? The only thing that mattered to me right then was to get the troubled player on the telephone, get him in my office, and get him the help he needed. I suddenly saw myself as a failure as a head coach. All the players knew about it, and I was too blind to see what was obvious to them. They had been looking to me to resolve a problem, and I was doing nothing about it. I felt stupid. All the signs had been there to see. I had rose-colored glasses on and couldn't see what was obvious to all the players. There are so many coaches, employees, parents, and friends who have been equally naive.

I immediately told my secretary, "Call ——— and tell him it's critical that he sees me immediately. Tell him I won't accept any excuse whatever."

He walked into my office the next day. I looked at him. He was the picture of confidence, even cocky, as he sat down. I decided to skip the small talk and go for the jugular vein. I said, "We're gonna talk for five minutes and what we're gonna talk about is your drug problem."

"Coach I——"

"Shut up. This is a five-minute conversation, and it's only one way! I'm the only one who's gonna talk. You're gonna listen. Lemme tell you this: it's my way or Trailway! If you don't listen to exactly what I tell you, you're outta here! I'm gonna cutcha! I'll putcha on waivers, and you're finished because I have all the evidence. I'm not even gonna display the evidence because this is not a court and it's not a trial. I *know* you're guilty. I *know* you have a drug problem. I *know* you have a chemical dependency problem. I thought for a long time maybe you weren't good enough, but you and I know that's not true.

"Now listen to me. You're going for an evaluation. My job is not to sit here and diagnose or moralize and try to find out why you would throw away your entire life. That's not my job. My job is to get you to the doctor. When he evaluates you, whatever he says, that's what you're gonna do!

"If you don't wanta do that, get out! I don't ever wanta see you again, and I ain't gonna worry about why. I'm gonna let you worry about why. It's time now, for the ball to be in your court. Everything will be very confidential. When I call the doctor's secretary, she'll never know your name. No one will know. You have to accept everything I'm telling you. You don't have a choice!"

By that time he was sweating. He was no longer cocky. He didn't know what to say. He had never in his life been put in a telephone booth like that. I knew I had to be tough. I knew I had to attack him as I just did because he wouldn't take me seriously otherwise. I took a deep breath and looked at him. The silence, as they say, was deafening. Then

I said softly, "I love ya and I wanta help ya. I wanta be involved with you and your family to bring your life back together. It's over. If you don't take this step, your pro football career is over. I know you're in the hole financially. What'll it be?"

I kept quiet then and took a deep breath, telling myself to stop talking now. What would he do? He didn't say anything. His head was still hanging down. I looked at him and waited. He slowly raised his head and looked at me. What would he do? Would he slug me? Would he turn his back on me and walk out? Time seemed to stop, my heart seemed to stop, my breathing seemed to stop. The whole world seemed to stop.

He moved slowly toward me, circled his arms around me and gave me a silent hug. Finally, almost in a whisper, he said, "Thanks, Coach Sam."

I stood there, saying to myself, *My God, my God, this is what life and football coaching are all about: motivating people to be their best.* This is not Don Shula being carried off the field after he won his first Super Bowl. This is not Chuck Noll being carried off the field in Los Angeles after winning his fourth Super Bowl. This is what coaching is all about to Sam Rutigliano, embracing a repentant guy who is sick, who needs help, who at one point was on top of the mountain with his dreams fulfilled, and now he's in my office, figuratively on his knees, frightened for his life, backed up to his own goal line, ready to do what he has to do to win again.

When he walked out of my office, I sat back and felt like I had just been through a championship football game or had just run a Boston Marathon. I was absolutely washed out, drained of all emotion. Yet it was an exhilarating feeling. A tremendous burden had just been lifted from me. I had learned that, when you confront addicts under the conditions we had, you don't give them a chance to say much. They're drug addicts. The first by-product of addiction is denial. The second is lying, pathological lying. It's almost like they're ventriloquists. The drug speaks for the drug addicts. It's a demon. It's out to kill the addicts. Robert Schuller was right when he said, "Tough times don't last, but tough people do."

# CHAPTER TWENTY-FIVE

# AFTERCARE

The only player to voluntarily step forward was the first one. Not one player confessed without being confronted. As we began to collect evidence from monitoring the players, I personally confronted each one. Even though the first player who volunteered to step forward spread the word within the team that the coach and the management could be trusted, still no other players would admit to using drugs. As most people know who work with addicts, they deny that they have a problem, and then they lie and lie and lie to cover up.

In the spring of 1982 I called one player after another into my office. Still they wouldn't volunteer to tell me they had a problem. Even after more players returned from the drug rehab center, they wouldn't trust anyone. Of course, they really didn't want to stop their habit. So we had to collect our evidence until we had an airtight case. I never zeroed in on a man unless I had a lot of evidence, which came from the equipment men, the trainer, the coaches, the doctor, and sometimes the wives of the players. The more drug addicts take drugs, the more chances they will take. Therefore, it was relatively easy to spot them by monitoring their behavior.

Our off-season training program started March 1 and lasted until July 1. The players worked on their individual skills, weight training, and body and strength development four out of five days each week. They went to training camp for thirty-five days where they got up at 6:30 in the morning and kept going until 11:00 P.M. It was intense. Then, in the regular season, they had to work every day except Tuesday. That's about as much strain as anybody can stand. During all those days, there was ample opportunity for all the monitors to watch the players.

But during off-season the players had plenty of time to lie around, watch TV, shoot baskets in a gym, and get bored. That's when the recovering addicts got in trouble. That's why we instigated the meetings to educate the straight players, in hopes of heading them off at the pass. Some of the straight players even came to the Inner Circle meetings. They told us they didn't do drugs but they had other problems they needed help with.

I didn't expect players to show up with the idea of helping, but that's what happened one day. I had invited two new men to the Inner Circle meeting. They were not users but had agreed to come. The meeting got started in the usual manner when a player stood and read the twelve steps used in Alcoholics Anonymous. Then the doctor stood and said, "Does anyone have anything to say?"

A player stood and said, "I'm still struggling with my marriage. My wife turns on that same old broken record about me caring more about football than her. Hey, when do I get any time to be with her? I'm always here."

After we talked about that problem for a while, another player said, "I've got a problem with my former drug dealer. He keeps calling me. Won't let me alone. Keeps tempting me."

Still another player said, "I'm not working in the off-season, and I can't handle my idle time."

One of the most shocking things I heard came from a player who said, "I'm livin' with my parents, tryin' to stay clean, right? Can you believe this? They're users! How am I gonna stay off the stuff with them smokin' joints all the time? I can't get them to stop. I can't get them to go see the right people. It's like I'm sittin' on top of a keg of dynamite."

A string of problems surfaced and were shared openly. Then toward the end of the meeting, someone asked the two visitors what they thought about what they had heard.

One man stood. I didn't know what to expect. I did know that he wasn't a user and that he was a Christian. He said, "Where's God in all this? What are you guys gonna do when you leave the team? Right now you've got all kinds of reinforcements. But what happens to you when you stop playing football and go out into the real world? You've got Art Modell who pays for your drug screen, pays for the doctor, pays for you to go to the drug rehab centers, pays for these meetings, pays Calvin Hill's salary, pays Paul Warfield's salary, pays Sam Rutigliano. Where you gonna be when you leave here? Where you gonna find this kind of support group? How are you gonna make it? There's only one way you can do it."

All eyes were glued on him. Several of the guys said, "What're you talkin' about, man?"

He said, "There's only one answer. If you get hurt in this business, you're finished. This is a fragile business. You can get cut tomorrow. You can get hurt tomorrow. Your career can end tomorrow. You're not gonna play football the rest of your life. Some day you're gonna be thirty-two years old and then you've got your whole life ahead of you. You've got forty or fifty more years to go. You've gotta deal with sobriety the rest of your life. What kind of Higher Power do you have to help you?" He looked at the men. Then his voice softened, "I'll tell you how you can do it."

The room was as silent as a woods before daybreak. Everyone stared at him. Here was a guy offering to share a secret that might take the drug monkey off their backs. Here was a player everybody respected. He had credibility. Everybody knew he wasn't a user. He had come with an answer—the Answer. And then he said, "It's Jesus Christ. Only your commitment to the Savior will bring you through the rest of your life."

The other man stood and said much the same thing. We didn't set it up. They weren't users, but they were high on Christ and it showed. The players' curiosity was aroused. They wanted to know more. What the two men had said fit right in, especially with one of the twelve points of Alcoholics Anonymous. Each user would admit he could no longer control his life. The visitors were offering a new hope.

Tom Petersberg, the spiritual leader of the group, immediately showed the Scriptures that supported what the men had said. From that point on, the Inner Circle really took off. Soon about six of the guys and their wives started a Bible study at one of their homes. Tom Petersberg led a Bible study in the locker room on Wednesdays right after practice. We got the Browns to buy pizzas to serve when the study was over. Soon we had thirty-five to forty players, and some of the wives and girlfriends joined us. We started having chapel both at home and away. On the road, the players attended a chapel service about four hours before kickoff. Thirty or forty people, including wives and children, went to the services. People were growing spiritually. If it took a pepperoni pizza to get some people to hear God's Word, then it was all worthwhile.

As I look back on it, I realize that I wasn't the one who started all this spiritual stuff at the Browns. It wasn't even Tom Petersberg, the chaplain. It was God who intervened.

Things really got moving after that. The Inner Circle grew. I was elated. One day I said to the doctor, "Isn't it great the way things are progressing?"

He said, "That's what I'm worried about. Things are going *too* well."

"Whattaya mean, Doc?"

"I don't hear the players arguing or disagreeing or trying to cover up with lies. Things are too quiet. I'm worried."

I said, "Aw, come on, Doc. This program isn't as difficult as I thought it was going to be. Very frankly, I think you're overreacting."

"Maybe, but I don't think so."

We parted that day, and I kept wondering why he was worried. I didn't have long to wait before I found out.

A few days later, the Inner Circle came together for a regular meeting. Calvin Hill was there along with Paul Warfield, Tom Petersberg, the doctor, and me. As soon as everyone sat down, the doctor threw a bomb into our midst. "We've got a problem. All the urine screens are clean. No way can all you guys be clean. There's no trace of marijuana or cocaine in any of the specimens."

I said, "What are you saying, Doc? That they're faking the specimens?"

"Yes."

"Are you sure?"

"Yes."

"What's the matter with you guys? Do you actually want to commit suicide? Do you think this whole thing is a big joke? What kind of fools do you think we are?" Calvin Hill and Paul Warfield were even more explosive. We all began yelling at the guys.

I got as angry as I've been in years. I felt like the guy who discovers his wife has been cheating on him and everybody has known except him. I screamed at them, "Whattaya think you're doin'? I'm sick of you guys. I'm ready to throw all of you out in the street. I'm ready to quit. The newspapers were right when they said we were running a half-way house for rich, spoiled brats. They were right when they said, 'We don't want the Inner Circle. We want the Winners' Circle.' Look at you, all of you sitting here with your heads down, like a bunch of puppies who just got caught urinating on the carpet! I feel like pullin' the pin from a grenade and tossin' it right in the middle of all you guys! Look at yourselves! You can't even look us in the eyes. I feel like tellin' all you guys to get outta my life, get outta the Browns, get outta football! You really can't change the spots on a leopard! There's no way in the world I want to be involved with you guys any longer!"

Several of the players spoke at once, "Coach, we didn't mean to——"

"I don't wanta hear your excuses. Excuses are like elbows, everybody's always got a couple. You've made us all look like fools. We made all this effort. Art Modell has spent thousands of dollars. Whattaya think about the other players? They think we've been mollycoddling you guys. They think we're bogus. The media people think we're nuts. Some of the other coaches are calling me and criticizing what we're doing. They're saying, 'It ain't gonna work.'

"Now it looks like all of them were right and we're a bunch of patsies. How does it feel to make me look like a patsy, huh? How could you do this? We're tryin' to give this idea substance. The only substance we have right now is chemical! It's like building a house. We got the foundation and then the building itself, and then we discover that the foundation was wrong." I stopped for breath, and it hit me that I was moralizing. "Whoa, time-out! I'm moralizing! You guys——" My voice trailed off. I looked at the doctor and was shocked at what I saw. He was smiling, for cryin' out loud!

He said, "These things are going to happen."

No one spoke for a few seconds. Presently I said softly, "Ya know something, you guys? I love ya. Yeah, that's right, I love ya. What we need to do right now is close ranks. We need to put our arms around each other and start all over again."

The doctor looked at the guys and said, "The drug screen is an integral part of treatment. From now on, Paul Warfield and Calvin Hill are gonna watch you to make sure there's integrity in the tests. We're gonna have a drug screen every Monday and Thursday or Friday. We're gonna watch you guys. If that's the way it has to be, then we're gonna do it. You guys have to stay clean. You don't have the ability to resist drugs on your own until you've gone at least a year or a year and a half of being drug-free. The only way you can stay drug-free is to be accountable. You can't shoulder this by yourselves. All the promises in the world aren't gonna get it done without accountability. Right now you guys are cheating because you're not drug-free. You guys know how it is when you're dirty. You lie, you cheat, you cover up. I'll tell you what, you're all gonna be tested today. You better confess now while you've got a chance. If you don't, we'll get rid of you tomorrow!"

Our doctor was mild-mannered, but he was tough. He told it straight. We couldn't have made it without him.

And so we had in place a very expensive, very effective program that covered all the bases: prevention, intervention, and aftercare. Anonymity was essential. But we had no idea just how difficult it was going to be to maintain it.

# CHAPTER TWENTY-SIX

# THE CODE
# OF SILENCE

In Italian the word is *omerta*. Silence. You can make a lot of mistakes in what you say, but you rarely make a mistake by keeping silent. We had a code of silence within the Inner Circle. We knew there would be leaks here and there. Loose lips sink ships. Other players were going to find out who the members of the Inner Circle were. We allowed any player to attend the meetings. However, each member of the Inner Circle vowed never to divulge names or verify names in response to questions. Without proof, then, the media people couldn't reveal names. The integrity of the people involved in the Inner Circle would remain intact.

Early on, we had tremendous pressure from the media to reveal players' names. When Peter Axthelm wrote an article in *Newsweek*, I told a lot about how members of the press, particularly in Cleveland, were very much against me and what I was trying to do. As recently as the summer of 1986, after Don Rogers's tragic death, the *Cleveland Plain Dealer* still took shots at me. It seemed ludicrous. The Browns organization had a working drug prevention, intervention, and aftercare program, five years ahead of all the rest of the professional sports fraternity. Many of them were only in the early stages of trying to deal with a problem that simply would not go away.

I remember when a writer from the *Plain Dealer* came to me and said a woman had sent him a letter containing all the names of the Inner Circle members. His boss also came to me and said he needed to write about all the Inner Circle members. He said the story wouldn't hurt the players and it would be a good story in Cleveland. I told him there was no way I would give him permission to publish any names. I simply told him that his list of names was inaccurate. He wanted to know if some of the names were correct. I answered again that the list was inaccurate. I said I would ask the Inner Circle members if they were willing to have their names published with stories about their problems. To a man, they wanted no part of it.

Every player was deathly afraid of being told to take a walk. Many of the players wanted to go on into the business world. It wouldn't help them to be presented to the public as drug addicts. They had beaten the demon. They had knocked it off their backs. They wanted to forget it and get on with their lives and, perhaps, stay in Cleveland. Or if they wanted to go back to their respective hometowns and become coaches, the doors might be slammed in their faces. What good could come of newspaper stories about their sordid pasts now that they were on the road to full recovery? I'm glad to say that most of those men are living well-adjusted lives now and they still protect one another's identity. The code of silence.

But the media kept hounding me. The pressure from the *Cleveland Plain Dealer* was intense. The reporters threatened to publish their list of names with or without our permission. I told them again that the list was inaccurate. Then I arranged a meeting with the newspaper people, Art Modell, and me. Art told them strongly that they could never legitimately publish those names because they were inaccurate. Then they tried to get us to admit that some of the names were correct. We repeated the chorus that the names were inaccurate. *Omerta!* The pressure was intensified until Art Modell finally told them that there would be a tremendous lawsuit if they printed the names. If they published inaccurate names, their newspaper would no longer have the credibility to cover the Cleveland Browns. Art Modell was strong and the *Cleveland Plain Dealer* backed off—but they never forgot it. Some of those same people still take shots at me whenever they can. But I understand that reporters have to do their jobs and newspapers have to sell papers. I support the idea of a free press 100 percent. I'll give them credit; they tried everything they could think of to get those names. If they had succeeded, life could have been even more difficult for some of those players.

Look at the case of Dwight Gooden, the young pitcher for the New York Mets. At nineteen years of age, he was Rookie of the Year. At age 20, he won the Cy Young Award. At age 21, he went to the World Series and the Mets won the world championship. At age 22, he reported in because of illegal drug use. He then went to a drug rehab center somewhere in New York. Everyone saw him on a national television newscast being led away. A crowd had gathered there, some cheering, some booing. Incredibly, they were asking Dwight for his autograph.

Can you picture that young guy sometime in the future as he stands on the mound facing a batter? Suppose it's the bottom of the ninth inning with runners on second and third and he throws a home-run pitch to lose the game. No pitcher can win every game. He's not gonna strike everybody out. He'll have his highs and lows. Now I ask you, how does a young pitcher deal with a New York crowd in New York City? For that matter, how will he deal with every other city the team visits? Anytime he does something wrong on the mound he'll hear the fans talking about his drug habit, one way or the other, sooner or later. They'll love him only as long as he wins. As Walter Cronkite used to say, "And that's the way it is."

Wouldn't it have been better if there had been prevention and intervention so that he could have dealt with his problem anonymously? I can't help wondering what might have happened if someone like Dwight Gooden could have talked with some of the Inner Circle players. It's only conjecture, of course, but any thoughtful person can see it might have helped.

It's very interesting for me to compare what happened in Cleveland through the Inner Circle and the rest of professional sports. To my knowledge, there isn't one program in professional sports today that has the same type of aftercare. Yes, there's prevention. Yes, there's intervention. Yes, there's education. But where's the aftercare?

Look at what's happening in professional basketball as of this writing. Walter Davis, a great young player on the Phoenix Suns basketball team, is now going to a drug rehab center for the second time. Young players might possibly be indicted, according to the newspapers. Who knows? Maybe some of them wanted to quit but wouldn't step forward for fear of getting fired. Retribution is real, of course. Many people are hardnosed about players who use drugs. It's a lot of trouble to contend with players like that, no question about it. In my opinion the drug problem isn't going to disappear by itself. Professional sports management is going to have to face it sooner or later, like cancer. The sooner you detect it, the better the chances for recovery. Which is more cost effective in the long run?

How could Dwight Gooden's addiction have come as a shock to anyone? The guy didn't win a game in the playoffs or in the World Series, and he even missed the victory parade in New York City. How could a World Series player miss the parade in New York City? Wasn't anybody paying attention when he was arrested for drunken driving and had an altercation with a police officer? It was "boys will be boys" time again. A baseball team plays 162 regular games each year. If there had been a monitoring program, wouldn't someone have noticed if a player was "acting funny"?

In the Inner Circle we had all the structure right there. First, prevention, then monitoring, then intervention, then confrontation, then whisk them off to the doctor for evaluation, then off to the drug rehab center, then back to the team and ninety meetings the first ninety days back—meetings with the Inner Circle, meetings with Narcotics Anonymous at the Cleveland Clinic, weekly meetings with the doctor and two drug screens each week with someone watching the specimen being voided. Tough love! A guy can't screw up! But if he *does* screw up after all that aftercare effort, you gotta get rid of him. The player knows that if he takes one step back, it's all over. At that point we told him to put up or shut up. You're going our way or Trailway.

At Cleveland, we had a chance to monitor players. Art Modell was willing to pay for everything. He should get some kind of medal for what he's done to combat drugs. I've seen the system work. Why can't other teams do the same? Why won't other teams listen to Art Modell, to me, to Carl Eller, to the doctor? I don't know the answer to that. I've heard people in baseball say that the drug problem is waning. Then a Dwight Gooden story hits the papers.

In basketball some say there is a system that encourages drug-using players to come forward. But after they have come forward and completed treatment in a drug rehab center, there is no aftercare. If they continue their use of drugs, eventually they're suspended for life. What is a guy thirty-two years of age going to do after playing sports all his life and finding himself kicked out on the sidewalk? He goes from making $1 million a year to nothing. What's he gonna do? He's not going to get much sympathy anywhere.

Just recently Larry Bethea, the number-one draft choice of the Dallas Cowboys, who played at Michigan State, committed suicide in Virginia. He blew his head off! A year ago he stole $64,000 from his own mother. He was arrested. Somewhere along the line he may have been saved. What happened to Don Rogers? What happened to Len Bias? Many people are totally unsympathetic toward highly paid athletes who go astray. They say those athletes made their own choices. That's true. Am I my brother's keeper? Yes, the invasion of privacy is there, but we could, somehow, some way, save the lives of some young people. There *must* be a middle ground that would include prevention, intervention, and aftercare. I don't see this happening often enough in professional sports in America. Nobody seems to want to talk about how prevalent drugs are on the professional sports scene in America. Talk about the code of silence!

Speaking of silence, I should have extended my silence to other areas of my life. There came a time when I should have taken my father's advice and said nothing because of "the people in the hallway."

# CHAPTER TWENTY-SEVEN

# THE PEOPLE IN THE HALLWAY

In the spring of 1984 I discovered that one of my assistant coaches was undermining me behind my back. As an assistant coach, you can make mistakes, but you'd better be on the same page with the head coach. That includes loyalty. There is no room whatsoever for a staff person who is disloyal. Loyalty goes up the organization, and it goes down the chain of command. If there's a weak link in the chain, the entire chain is weak and will ultimately break if put under too much strain. Loyalty is the glue holding the coaching staff together. If we disagree in staff meetings, we talk about the issue until we reach a consensus. Then we put our personal feelings aside, pull together, and never look back. Football is a *team* effort. You can disagree but don't be disagreeable.

One day a well-respected player came into my office. He had been an outstanding player for the Browns for many years. He's out of football now, but he has my loyalty for life. He had the guts to tell me something I didn't want to hear. When parents first hear their children are using drugs, the first reaction is to deny the truth of it. I really respected this man, and when he spoke to me, I was shocked by what he said.

"Coach, one of your staff is torpedoing you behind your back. I thought you should know before the guy screws up the team. He's bad-mouthing you in front of a lot of the players, including me."

"Thanks. It's sad to hear this, but I'll look into it right away." I checked with several people, and they verified the story. I took my time, thinking it over fully before I decided what to do. My first stop was at Art Modell's office. When I told him what I had learned, he was angry.

"Sam, get rid of him right away. I don't want him around any longer. I especially don't want him around during the player draft. Get rid of him. I'm behind you 100 percent of the way."

The next day I called the coach into my office. I said, "I found out from reliable sources that you're undermining me, and I want you to clear out your desk and leave right away. There's nothing to discuss. You're through here. I could never feel the same about you after this. I want you to go to your office right now, pack, and leave. You're no longer on the coaching staff of the Cleveland Browns." I walked behind him and watched while he gathered up his belongings, and I waited until he left. It was a sad and difficult thing to do, but it had to be done. This episode was a foreboding of what 1984 was going to be like. Friends are made by many acts, lost by one.

The preseason games brought no improvement to my mood. To top it off, Cody Risien, who has since that time gone to the Pro Bowl, went down with a knee injury in the last preseason game, which we played in Philadelphia. Cody's injury was so severe we lost him for the entire season. Not only did we have to juggle the lineup, we had a new quarterback in Paul McDonald. Brian Sipe was gone to the USFL with Don Trump's New Jersey Generals. Paul needed those offensive linemen who formed a barbed-wire fence in front of him. The most important thing an NFL quarterback needs is pass protection. Although Paul didn't have a good year, one of the reasons for his poor showing was his lack of pass protection.

We lost our first game to Seattle. We didn't just lose it. We lost it so bad we couldn't find it. But that was just the beginning of the massacre. We lost seven close games. But a loss is a loss is a loss, even if by only 1 point. We lost 20–17 to the Los Angeles Rams, a game in which Paul threw an interception that became a touchdown. We lost 29–14 to the Denver Broncos, another game in which Paul threw an interception for a touchdown. We beat Pittsburgh at Cleveland Municipal Stadium, and it looked like we were back on track. Then we went to Kansas City where Paul threw four interceptions in the second half! We lost that game 10–6. We lost to New England 17–16; Paul threw an interception on their 15-yard line in the final minute of the game that took away our field-goal attempt and a probable win. Then we lost to the New York Jets, the New England Patriots, and the Bengals. Every one of them beat us by the closest margin.

The pivotal game, as far as my future was concerned, was with the New England Patriots, a game we lost by 1 point, 17–16. It was the sixth game of the year. I felt like throwing up. My blood pressure must have been up. If anybody had measured my anxiety level, it would have gone off the chart. Picture this. We're on their 15-yard line with about a minute to go in the game. The score is 17–16. We're just where I want to be. Just a field goal is all we need. McDonald has used up our last time-out. I call one more pass to get a little closer for the field-goal attempt by Matt Bahr. He had missed one earlier from that same spot.

My call was a mistake. In that situation anything can happen: a fumble when the center snaps the ball, a fumble by the quarterback, or an interception. Other than that there's nothing to worry about! When you're that close, you hunker down, kick the field goal, and let it fly. Then you're ahead 19–17 with only a few seconds left to worry about. You then kick off to New England, and they have about fifty seconds to score. Great odds for us if we had kicked the field goal. You play the percentages.

But I gambled. Gambling is fine in a football game, but you've got to know when to do it. This was not the time to do it. Paul McDonald dropped back in a perfect pocket with perfect pass protection and threw a perfect interception! It's easy now for me to say he never should have tried to force the ball. He should have thrown the ball away. Only if you need a crucial first down in situations like that do you try to force the ball. But otherwise, play the percentages. We weren't really that far away, and we should have gone for the field goal. I've dreamed about that mistake many nights. But in fairness to Paul, he was a young, inexperienced quarterback, and after all, I called the play. It was my mistake. Experience is a wonderful thing. It enables you to recognize a mistake when you make it.

After the game I dragged myself into the locker room. We were 1–5. We should have been 2–4. It wouldn't have been so bad that year because everybody in our division was struggling. We still could have been alive, even at the halfway mark, with a record of 4–4 or 3–5. There was always hope from week to week until the game with New England. We blew it. I blew it. I told the players in the locker room that I blew it. For the first time I was so upset with myself that I didn't take time to pray privately. I had to get to the press conference, knowing what was awaiting me there. Those guys would have me for lunch. Sometimes it's important to be honest, and sometimes it's important not to say anything. As my dad always said, "Whenever you have an opportunity to keep your mouth shut, take advantage of it." I wish I could have remembered that during the press conference.

Marty Schottenheimer, our assistant coach at the time, came to my office after the game and said, "Sam, don't get down on yourself. You're human. Everybody makes mistakes. You're only human." I always appreciated Marty's comments, but I was the one who had to face Art Modell in a few minutes. A man may make a mistake, but he isn't a failure until he starts blaming someone else.

As it turned out, I broke my own cardinal rule and spoke out when I was under great stress. It happened after the press conference when Barb and I went to Art Modell's office. Barb tried her best to calm me down before going into the lion's den, but I wouldn't listen to her. I knew it would be far worse than the press conference. I stormed out of the locker room and headed for Art's office with Barb trailing me, trying to head me off in the hallway. I wouldn't be stopped. I would face him, confess it was my fault, and take my lumps. I didn't think; I didn't pray. A terminal case of self-pity had already set in, and it was fatal.

When I walked into Art's office, the only thing missing was a body in a coffin. It was like a funeral. Art and Pat Modell were there along with the entire management team. It was a full quorum of pallbearers. Barb and I sat down. She kept nudging me to shut up, but I wouldn't. She wanted me to go through minimum cordiality requirements dictated by common courtesy and split that place. She wanted me to say, "Sorry we didn't win. It was my fault. Paul never should have thrown the interception. Let's all get a good night's rest. I'll look at the film and call you tomorrow. I'll stop by your house tomorrow evening, and we'll watch the first half of the 'Monday Night Football' game together. Then we can talk about it. I'll bring a pizza!" That's what I *shoulda* said. Shoulda, woulda, coulda.

What I *did* say was this: "Art, I lost that game. It wasn't Paul Mc-Donald's decision to pass instead of kick; it was mine. I never should have called the pass. I should have lined up and kicked the field goal." I noticed everyone in the room focusing on me, listening intently. I felt myself getting more and more emotional. My self-pity quotient was exploding off the chart! I said to Art, "Listen, if you wanta fire me right now, I won't hold you to our new contract. You can fire me right now if you want." I was into it up to my neck, and I could see Barb shrug in desperation. But I wouldn't stop. I wouldn't even slow down. I grabbed a piece of paper off Art's desk and ripped it apart. "Art, if you want to tear up my contract, you won't have any responsibility after today!" I looked at Barb again, and she was stunned, speechless.

The one thing I can say in my own defense about that pitiful scene is that no one in the room with me really knew what I was feeling just then. None of them were coaches. No way could they identify with me. I decided later, when my tongue caught up with my mind, that they viewed my outburst as a sign of weakness. It was ironic. How many times I had been with Art when he was so down he wanted to sell the team. He wanted out. That's when I had encouraged and comforted him. I looked at the others, some of whom I had helped in the past. They looked like my pallbearers, peering down at me in a coffin. It was apparently too late for comfort because nobody comforted me. They just stared at me as if I had AIDS. What I saw on their faces was the expression people have when they visit someone in intensive care. But this disaster was my own fault. When you lose a game, it's the coach's fault. That's the way it is. Only Barb would still love me after that day.

But Art came through for me—at the moment at least. He jumped up out of his chair and almost yelled, "I'm not John Mecon or Bob Irsay! I don't fire coaches in midstream! That's a cop-out! We're a family, and we're in this together! We'll just figure a way out."

Pat Modell got up and put her arms around Barb and said, "Listen, Barb, there's nothing for you to worry about."

Presently everything calmed down, and we left.

In the car Barb said, "That was a mistake. I can't believe you would open yourself up like that in front of those people. They don't understand. You shouldn't have said anything. The only people who really understand are the coaches who walk the sidelines. Those people are going to view that emotional display as weakness. They're going to say, 'Sam is coming apart at the seams. The pressure is getting to him. Sam is going to lose control of this football team. I don't think we can win with him, and we'd better make a change if he doesn't turn this thing around in the next couple of weeks.'"

My little Barb was absolutely right. Like Sgt. York, she hit the bull's-eye. My outburst may not have changed things in the long run, but I never should have opened myself up to that entire group. I should have spoken privately to Art and no one else. They thought I was going wacko.

Within the next two years, I heard everyone who had been in that room say, "We did it for Sam. He was coming apart. We did it in the best interests of the Cleveland Browns." Dad was right. I should have kept my mouth shut after that game. I lost my close, one-on-one contact with Art that day, a common bond that had started the night I met Art and Pat. It was the same current of understanding that had brought us through many other bad times. But the electricity had short-circuited and was gone. I had allowed the people in the hallway to come between us. The people who were there that day sat together in the luxury loges. They can all sit there and second-guess the coach every game. It's not the owner who usually fires you; it's the people in the hallway, the ones who have the king's ear. He pulls the trigger, but they line up the rifle.

# CHAPTER TWENTY-EIGHT

# FOLLOW THE FOLLOWER

**I**n the draft of 1984 the Cleveland Browns selected Don Rogers number one. Don was an All-American free safety from UCLA. He was a big, strong tackler with tremendous athletic skills, and he had all the prerequisites you look for in a free safety. A free safety is the last line of defense. He's the guy who has to make the big plays. He must be a great tackler because if he misses a tackle, the next place the runner crosses is the goal line. A free safety is the hub of the defense, and all the other defensive backs and linebackers are spokes in the wheel. He has to have superior intelligence because he makes all the last-second changes on the line of scrimmage. He directs and orchestrates the strong safety, both cornerbacks, and all the linebackers in the underneath coverage.

When I sent Marty Schottenheimer out to California to look at film and to study Don Rogers, we already knew that he had all the physical skills. The thing we were most concerned about was whether or not he could be an immediate starting player in the NFL. Even though UCLA is the highest level of college football, there is a very big difference between college and pro football. At UCLA a player might play against a Dan Fouts once or twice, but in the NFL he would be up against Dan Fouts thirteen or fourteen times. All the while, Dan Fouts and players of his caliber are getting better and better each year. So we drafted Don Rogers, but we watched him very carefully during the entire training camp to see if he was going to be able to handle all the mental challenges a free safety would face in the NFL.

Now that we have hindsight, we had the opportunity to draft Louis Lipps instead of Don Rogers, and the press never let us forget it. We picked Don Rogers before Pittsburgh picked Louis Lipps, a man who became an instant superstar, a punt returner, and a Pro Bowl receiver.

He could have helped the Browns very much. As I've worked games in Pittsburgh for NBC, I've often appreciated his great talent. The press put tremendous pressure on us after the 1984 season because of the success of Louis Lipps.

In the 1984 training camp I asked Marty Schottenheimer repeatedly how Don Rogers was coming along. Don was a primary project for Marty, whose answer was always the same, "He's really picking up everything we're trying to do. He's mentally alert, he understands what people are trying to do to him, he understands it in meetings, in individual and group practices, and in the scrimmages. I've had no problem with him in the preseason games."

During the time I coached him, up until the infamous Cincinnati game, Don Rogers' talents on the field were obvious. He played well with Al Gross, the strong safety, with Hanford Dixon and Frank Minnifield, our two cornerbacks, and with Clay Matthews and Chip Banks, our two linebackers. It seemed like he had played with them for an extended period of time.

But let's go back to the first time I met Don Rogers. I was very impressed with him and the way he looked me in the eye. I had read and heard what other people had said about him and I had talked with him on the telephone, but I wanted to see him face-to-face. When you draft a guy in the first round these days, you'd better know everything about him, including his Social Security number, height, weight, speed, background, former trainers, coaches, assistant coaches, teachers, high-school coaches, and even relatives. The research is exhaustive. It's a tremendous investment, and you just can't afford to make a mistake in the first round. The first-round draft choice has to be able to start, have a positive impact on the team, and help you right away.

We had a hole at free safety. Don Rogers filled that hole. Don had a tremendous Rose Bowl game that year when UCLA won in January of 1984. We were very pleased with our draft choice. I was pleased with him as a man, somehow, because he looked me right in the eye and gave me a good, strong handshake. I simply had a good feeling about Don from the first time I met him. The vibes were there. He had all the qualities, but he also had that little extra: he had an intense desire to be the best.

Ken Easley is probably the best strong safety in the NFL today. He's the All-Pro strong safety from Seattle who also played at UCLA. When I first met Don Rogers, I knew he wanted to be like Ken Easley. He had emulated Easley at UCLA, and he wanted to emulate Easley's professional attainments. When we drafted Don, the United States Football League was still intact. The team in Phoenix, the Arizona Wranglers coached by George Allen, also had the rights to Don Rogers. They made a public statement after we drafted Don that they were going to go all out to sign him.

When Don came to talk with us in Cleveland, Paul Warfield and Calvin Hill picked him up at the airport and drove him to the stadium. He talked with the press, Art Modell, Ernie Accorsi, Kevin Byrne (the publicist), and me. We had dinner with him and all the other draft choices. Helping us host these men were former Browns stars Lou Groza, Dante Lavelli, Reggie Rucker, and Ron Bolton. We wanted to introduce them to the Cleveland community, the Browns, the stadium, the training camp, and the town itself. It would be a place where they might well play for ten years and raise their families. Many ex-Browns players stay in Cleveland after they retire from football.

I said to Don, "I know there's a bidding war and Phoenix is interested in you. But remember, of all the people you've met, I'm the guy you're gonna go into the bunker with. I'm the guy you're gonna go into the foxhole with. I'm the guy you're gonna have to be involved with one-on-one daily. The reason you're here is because you're a great football player. Your number-one goal is to continue to ascend as a football player.

"Remember this: don't ever let a third party communicate to me. I don't wanta communicate through your agent. I will never allow an owner, a newspaperman, or anybody in management to communicate to you what I want you to know. We drafted you number one, and that has to be a clear indication of how great a player we think you are. We've done our homework. If you come in here and get involved in our off-season program for about six to eight weeks before training camp starts and you're religious about that, I can guarantee you, with the ability you have right now, going into training camp with that head start, you're gonna be a starter this year. I can guarantee that only if you fulfill your part of it. But don't play games with your agent. I'm asking you to come in, even if you don't sign."

We wanted him to know about Cleveland firsthand. We didn't want his agent to draw pictures for him, whispering to him, subtracting, adding, and multiplying what Cleveland was all about. He could see for himself, and that's why we took him everywhere and had him meet everybody. I wanted to clear the air with Don, and I did the same with all the draft choices from top to bottom. Everybody, including Marty Schottenheimer, Bill Davis, director of player personnel, Tom Miner, the West Coast scout, and me, agreed that Don Rogers was top drawer. We had a consensus. We simply had to eliminate the possibility of a mistake with a number-one draft choice. We all agreed that Don could be our starting free safety.

And so, when I first met Don and he looked me in the eye, he said, "Coach, I want to play pro football and I want to be a great player and I want to play here for the Cleveland Browns."

The bidding war began. Ernie Accorsi's primary responsibility with the Browns organization was to sign players. Although signing players was not my responsibility, I became involved and went all out to let Don see who and what we really were. We had become friends when he visited us. That way, no agent could come in and start an adversarial relationship. Already Don had friends in Cleveland before his agent arrived on the scene.

We signed Rogers and had a press conference, with tables and chairs, in the left-field grass of Cleveland Municipal Stadium on a sunny June day. That day I had the same strong, good feeling about Don. At the press conference he looked at me and smiled as if to say, "Coach, I told you I'd sign with Cleveland." Don's agent, Steve Arnold, was there from New York, and everybody was happy, including Arnold. We simply had no big problems with either the Phoenix team or the agent. That showed me the kind of guy Rogers was. He was committed to the best and to being the best. He wanted to play in the NFL, he wanted to reach the summit, he wanted to play in a stadium where some of the greatest players in the history of the game played. Otto Graham, Jim Brown, Lou Groza, Dante Lavelli. You could see it in Don Rogers's eyes. You could almost feel it all around you in that huge stadium. Don was on his way to joining those legendary players. I could just feel it. Cleveland has been and still is the flagship of the NFL fleet as evidenced by the number of Hall of Fame players.

Sometimes when I drive my car and stop for a red light, my mind goes back to the day in the stadium when we signed Don and he shook my hand and was so thrilled to be a pro football player. Then when the light turns green and I move on, I say to myself, *My gosh, what a tragic waste of a twenty-three-year-old, vibrant young man.* That was the beginning with Don Rogers.

In our many meetings, at first, Don always made eye contact with me. He never looked away, and he always smiled. He always seemed glad to be there because he loved to play football. But then, I can remember my father saying to me, "Show me your friends and I'll show you what you are and what kind of job your mother and I did in raising you." Don's directness and ability to look people in the eye were very important to me. I even looked players in the eye when we lost games. I could distinguish the guys who were involved more in themselves than in the program as team members. Don wasn't self-centered, even though he did have his individual goals as everybody should have.

But something happened in training camp when the veterans first reported. I could sense something was different about Don. I coached him during the first eight games in 1984. I was fired after that. During those games, however, I discovered that Don Rogers was a follower. He desperately wanted to be accepted by his peers. A football team has a small group of negative people and a small group of positive ones. Don began to follow the negative ones. It was his choice. I wasn't the only one who saw that he wasn't keeping the best of company. There were comments in the newspapers about this after his death.

Coaches and owners can only do so much. Art Modell did far more than any owner, in my view, to discourage and control the terrible use of drugs on his football team. I can't imagine anyone doing more. He certainly did more than anyone had a right to expect. No matter what happened, he can surely hold his head high because of his tremendous efforts to deal with the problem. He gave me absolute and full support in my efforts.

Everybody seems to want the drug problem simply to go away, but it's like cancer. You cut it out of one location, and it turns up in another. Everybody knows how it spreads if it's ignored. We wanted our players to know how insidious drugs are. You can't ignore cancer or drugs. If they aren't detected early, they may spread and become fatal. We were interested in prevention in the case of the young players.

Each year since 1982 we talked to all our draft choices and free agents about drugs and alcohol. We wanted them to know where we stood and where the NFL stood on these issues. In 1984 I sat down with the entire group of draft choices and told them about the Inner Circle. I used this example repeatedly: "Caterpillars get in long lines and follow one another. An entomologist once put some caterpillars on the rim of a big flowerpot. Food and water were inside the flowerpot, and the caterpillars continued to circle around the food but did not break ranks to get it. They followed one another until they starved to death within sight of food. You guys are going to experience peer pressure like you never did before. There's as much difference between the college environment and the pro environment as there is between night and day. Besides, at college you were stars; here you're rookies. From now on, you'll make more of your own decisions than you have in your life. You'll have to decide what to have for breakfast, lunch, and dinner. You'll have to take care of your own laundry, your car, your choice of roommates. No longer are you in a controlled environment on a college campus."

Then Calvin Hill and Paul Warfield, along with members of the Inner Circle, talked to the young men as well. We were involved and committed to a program of prevention and intervention as well as cure. It was so much easier to prevent than to cure. I personally sat down with Don Rogers and discussed all these issues.

In January of 1984 I attended a big scouting meeting that involved all the NFL teams. They bring the top three hundred players in the USA to it and put the players through a series of skill tests while all the coaches and scouts observe. In addition, each player is examined thoroughly by doctors, including orthopedic surgeons. Each player's joints are checked carefully. Then comes a drug screen. Don Rogers passed that drug screen.

After that, back at home just prior to training camp, each player was screened again for drugs. We did this every year. Remember, we had checked Don's background in every possible way—including talking with Terry Donahue, his coach at UCLA. All the reports we had were absolutely conclusive that Don Rogers was clean. Prior to training camp, Don passed the drug screen, too.

Don Rogers, to me, was a tremendous football player and a great person. But as the veterans came into training camp, I watched to see which line of caterpillars Don would join. He wanted to be accepted. There's nothing wrong with that unless you get in the wrong line. I was disappointed and alarmed to notice that Don was keeping the wrong company.

Calvin Hill and Paul Warfield spent a lot of time with all the new players, including them in our weekly Inner Circle meetings so they could get a perspective from players who entered the league just as they had. Each year, a new crop of nouveau-riche rookies come into the league and fall in line with some of the older guys. They very much want to be accepted as friends by these veterans, these role models whose ability and attainments they admire so much. Remember, less than 1 percent of all football and basketball players in America make it into the professional ranks. That's tall company. It's a dream come true for them. They have finally arrived after years of toil.

When the rookie football player arrives at training camp, he enters into a Spartan life. He's up at 6:30 every morning, there's breakfast, then a meeting, then a practice. After lunch there's another meeting and another practice, then weight training and running. He takes a deep breath and goes to dinner in the cafeteria. After a half-hour rest, he goes to another meeting, which breaks at 10:30, followed by a snack of cookies, ice cream, and fruit. He grabs that and falls into bed in time for a coach's bed check at 11:00 P.M. The good news is that he's going to have to do it all over again the next day and the next and the next.

The veterans, on the other hand, have been through it all before. Some of these guys are cool. After the afternoon practice, they take a shower and go out for a couple of beers before dinner. Some folks might agree that there isn't much apparent harm in having a couple of beers before dinner, right? What about the rookies? Who are they watching? Who do they want to emulate? Who do they want to be friends with? I guarantee you, they're eager to be friends with the veterans. So what happens when a star athlete, one the rookie has watched on television in the past, one he can't believe he's on the same team with, invites the rookie to "go for a coupla beers" before dinner? He can't wait. He'd take a pay cut to be this veteran's friend. And that's how it sometimes starts. The rookie goes out with the veterans because he wants them to like him.

I used to watch for who came in late at dinnertime. We always checked, and each player had to be there. Soon after everyone else had started eating dinner, the long line of sheep would file in late, eager-eyed rookies following, just like the caterpillars. There's nothing wrong with "relaxing," but not every player goes out before dinner simply to relax. If the rookie follows the wrong line, it might ultimately lead to becoming so relaxed he's limp.

Then, something worse can happen. As the 1983 Inner Circle players said to me, "Coach, after our first game against Minnesota at the stadium, some of our players will be introduced to cocaine for the first time at a party." The Inner Circle guys actually told the young players it would happen and to be on guard for it. They told them why they had done it and how they began to hang out with the players who used drugs. They even began to hang out with drug dealers in places frequented by users and dealers. The Inner Circle members told them they absolutely had to drop their old "friends" and find new faces and new places. Otherwise, they went right back to their old habits. Some of the players argued that they could stay clean and still associate with users. The Inner Circle members and the doctor warned them it would be impossible to do that. Don Rogers came into the NFL in 1984, and two years later he was dead.

We saved eleven lives on the Cleveland Browns. They're viable football players who, by the grace of God, were saved from drug addiction. What did it? Comprehensive rehabilitation centers, aftercare, Narcotics Anonymous at the Cleveland Clinic, two drug screens each week, visits to the doctor once each week, attendance at the Inner Circle meetings fifty-two weeks a year, and involvement of their wives. Some of them had been at death's door, losing $3,000 to $4,000 a week. The program saved them. It worked because of one word. Art Modell, the doctor, Carl Eller, Calvin Hill, Paul Warfield, several others, and I *cared*.

They say, today, that the "Just Say No" advertisements on television are not enough. We proved that if you cared—and everybody did—you could intervene through tough love and drug screens and save people's lives. All of us experienced it together.

The "Just Say No" to drugs slogan is like trying to say no to food. It works until you're hungry. The demon drug is the culprit. We humans are too weak to battle things like that without a Higher Power. Christ was the Higher Power who helped the Inner Circle members with whom I worked to recover. Each of those individuals finally looked to Him for help after trying desperately in every other way to beat the drug habit. I know it's tough for an organization to lose someone like Don Rogers, but what's to prevent it from happening again? Don Rogers made his own choices. What he did was his own fault and no one else's. Drugs ended Don's career.

Because of drugs, a player runs the risk of ending his career quicker than if he blew out a knee. More than that, he can end his life. Bad knees don't kill players; drugs kill players. In this country, we spend millions of dollars to prevent knee injuries and to operate on and rehabilitate knees. If someone invents a device or mechanism to prevent a bad knee from stopping an athlete's career, he's gonna be a billionaire. Where are our priorities? I don't think owners, general managers, and coaches can say drug prevention isn't their responsibility. The Browns knew that because of the recovered addicts on their team.

Everybody except one kept his anonymity. The bond we made in 1981 is still intact at this writing. The code of silence. I still have writers trying to get the names of the Inner Circle guys out of me. I've never told anyone, and I'll go to my grave with my silence. But newspapers continue to publish stories of players allegedly involved with drugs, including some former Browns.

Some say the drug problem is diminishing. Most people simply want it to go away. How much more is it going to take to prove to professional sports organizations that we have a huge problem in America today? There is a natural human tendency to ignore problems if they are out of our individual sight or if they are too horrible to face.

The reason I feel so strongly about combating drugs is that I was so personally involved, right in the trenches of the drug war with the addicts. I saw the highs and lows, met with the wives, the girlfriends, and the children. I saw players struggle through the strike years, I heard all the stories about drug dealers threatening them to pay their drug bills, I saw them cry like babies, and I saw the fear in their eyes that I might finally give up on them and kick them out of football. That's what Carl Eller told me about. He actually hid his habit for thirteen years. He desperately wanted to confess, but he knew his career would be over if he did.

I went through all that with our players. I felt like a grieving father toward those guys. I was with them when they were on their knees, when they broke drug screens, and when we went one-on-one, nose-to-nose. I was the guy who was there with them during the high moments and the low ones. I was the guy who put my arms around the users and told them I loved them.

Sure I took a lot of flack from other people about being too soft with them, but it was my choice and I'd do it again. That's why I can say to Pete Rozelle of the NFL and David Stern of the NBA and Peter Ueberroth of baseball, "I know how important aftercare is to save somebody's life." Without aftercare, it doesn't do much good to send users to a thirty day drying-out program. Art Modell is the only owner, to my knowledge, who provides adequate aftercare.

Almost every week we read of a professional athlete getting busted, sometimes for the second or third time. It's a terrible kind of seesaw life. It takes a year to a year and a half of being clean to really beat the drug habit. The temptation is always there; the dealers are always there.

I remember a player involved in the Inner Circle who came back from a trip "dirty." He had been to two drug rehabilitation centers. I sensed in the meeting that he was lying through his teeth. He failed the drug screen. Because of the period of time he was with us, we should have thrown him out. Calvin Hill, Paul Warfield, Tom Petersberg, and I were all there. We had sort of a "Last Supper" meeting. I looked the guy right in the eye and said, "You have to go to a drug rehab center, and you have to go tomorrow. It's gonna be a lot tougher than any you ever went to before."

He said, "I'm not going."

I stared at him and said, "That's fine. But I want you to know right now that if you don't go tomorrow, you're finished with the Browns. You're out of the Inner Circle, and I won't protect you and you can go to your grave because of drug use. If you don't go, you're finished."

He didn't want to go, but we had all the power and we used it for his benefit. I gave him his choice. I also gave him an airline ticket and waited a few hours for his decision. He went. That same year, after a preseason game, that player's counselor from the drug rehab center was there. The player had beat the drug demon.

Looking back, I'm sure that confrontational meeting saved the player's life, and everybody in the Inner Circle knew it. Art Modell and other people in the organization were pleased about what we had done and what we had accomplished.

Since that time, I've learned a great secret. It's a mistake for me to expect any credit or gratitude because of the success of the Inner Circle program or of any other efforts to help people. It isn't due me. The credit and the gratitude should be directed to the Lord. That knowledge fulfills me now. What gnaws at me is that the tragedies continue.

In the sports section of *The Palm Beach Post* on Sunday, June 14, 1987, a column written by Victor Lee and Patrick McManamon included this paragraph: "Nine days after (Len) Bias died, Cleveland Browns defensive back Don Rogers died of a heart attack caused by cocaine. According to Dr. Joseph Pursch of the Family Care Clinic in Newport Beach, Calif., 157 other Americans died the same way in the nine days between Rogers' and Bias' deaths."

The writers listed a "Drug Involvement Chronology" of events that occurred in the time between the deaths of Len Bias and Don Rogers. They cited 120 arrests of athletes, including boxers and jockeys and even coaches, and six drug-related deaths. Besides Bias and Rogers, the "Chronology" noted many other well-known athletes: Dwight Gooden of the New York Mets; Olympic diver Greg Louganis; LaMarr Hoyt, a major-league baseball pitcher; Walter David, an All-Star guard for the Phoenix Suns; Gary McClain, Villanova's 1985 star guard on the 1985 NCAA championship team, who stated that he was high when his team visited the White House and President Reagan; All-American linebacker Brian Bosworth of the University of Oklahoma; Warren McVea, who played for the Cincinnati Bengals; and Lewis Lloyd and Mitchell Wiggins of the Houston Rockets. The list went on.

Any thoughtful person must realize that those who are caught represent only the tip of the iceberg. The number of drug users in the United States who have not been caught must be astronomical.

On the other hand, the number of truly outstanding players is not astronomical. There are a few who have been larger than life during my tenure as a coach. It's a pleasure for me to pay tribute to them in the next chapter.

# WINNERS MAKE PLAYS, LOSERS MAKE EXCUSES

In 1978 during my first year as head coach of the Cleveland Browns, we won our first three games against San Francisco, Cincinnati, and Atlanta. Next we were going to Pittsburgh. Both the Browns and the Steelers were undefeated, but the Three Rivers Jinx still hung over our heads. The Browns had never beaten the Steelers there. Pittsburgh was destined to go to the Super Bowl in 1979 and 1980. They were seemingly indestructible.

The Central Division of the American Football Conference was the toughest in football, and Pittsburgh was leading the pack. I was advised to arrange a transfer into another division! Chuck Noll was beginning to reap the rewards of all the seeds he had planted and nourished in building his team. They were in full bloom when I arrived in Cleveland in 1978.

Terry Bradshaw had linemen in front of him like Mike Webster, Jon Kolb, and Larry Brown. His receivers were John Stallworth and Lynn Swann. Franco Harris was at fullback. Four of those seven players—and perhaps all of them—will be in the Hall of Fame.

Defense featured Joe Greene and L. C. Greenwood as part of the Steel Curtain. Jack Lambert and Jack Ham were linebackers. Mel Blount and Donnie Shell were in the secondary. Joe Greene is already in the Hall of Fame, and a trio or all five of the remaining defense could make it, also. It was almost impossible to structure a game plan against such an imposing group. The offense could make the big play and also control the ball by running it.

Defensively, they could cover your receivers and that caused sacks. Or they could rush with their front four and cause turnovers. The linebackers were the best combination in football. They were fast enough to open-field tackle the best running backs in the NFL. They could cover the backs coming out of the backfield as pass receivers. They could blitz and totally disorient your offense. Sometimes I wondered if we were going to have to ask for volunteers to go to Pittsburgh. However, they brought out the best in us, and we played from locker room to locker room and laid it on the line. We rarely left anything on the field.

Many people have asked me how the Central Division of the National Football League could be the poorest division in the 1980s when it was the toughest in the 1970s. The answer is very simple. When you lose starting quarterbacks like Ken Anderson of Cincinnati, Ken Stabler and Dan Pastorini at Houston, Brian Sipe at Cleveland, and Terry Bradshaw at Pittsburgh, you simply cannot replace quarterbacks of that caliber overnight. You can develop all the other areas of your squad, but if you don't have the engineer, the quarterback, you're not going to the summit. There are no exceptions. You simply have to have a great quarterback to win in the National Football League. He's the problem solver. He finds a way to win. He directs, orchestrates, and leads the team. Always calm under attack, he trusts his natural ability. One of the keys is discipline. Young quarterbacks will run more than necessary because each week they see something new and things happen so fast in the pro game they don't have time to react. Once they accustom themselves to various coverages and blitzes, they will run less. There are many old *throwing* quarterbacks but no old *running* quarterbacks.

Quarterbacks should be in silent communication with the receivers. They become accustomed to the body language of each receiver. Timing is essential to the quarterback, and each receiver has a different gait. Read, recognize, and throw in rhythm. The quarterback must see the defense in slow motion. Field vision and awareness are important as he anticipates throwing the ball. I like a quarterback who can run away from the rush but then use his speed to find an open receiver. A quarterback must have a short memory and not torture himself with second thoughts. He must avoid peaks and valleys and play with consistency. Finally he senses and feels pressure. We call it survival intelligence. Dan Fouts has an uncanny ability to duck under pressure. Dan Marino moves up into the pocket when he senses pressure. There should be a special Hall of Fame for Fouts because he never played with a strong defense. Dan Marino cuts up defenses, and they don't even know they're bleeding.

As you review the past, you see Otto Graham, Johnny Unitas, Bart

Starr, and Terry Bradshaw. Championships are what really count when you judge the great ones. Otto Graham won a championship every year he was a quarterback for the Cleveland Browns. I once spoke with Dr. Ippolito, the team doctor for the Browns for over forty years, who said, "I put thirty-six stitches in Otto's mouth at the half and told him he shouldn't play the second half. He said to me, 'I don't play with my mouth. I play with my mind and my body.'" A lot of quarterbacks would miss thirty-six games with that many stitches in their mouths. Otto Graham not only won games; he won championships. He has to be considered one of the greatest quarterbacks of all time. Think of how little money he played for in comparison to the salaries of today.

I can remember talking to Stan Jones, now a defensive line coach for the Denver Broncos, who said to me, "I played for the Chicago Bears for twelve years. I was an All-Pro offensive guard and an All-Pro defensive tackle. I made $100,000—but it took me twelve years to make it!" It's absolutely absurd to think about the salaries of today as compared to those of people like Otto Graham.

As an assistant coach, I was fortunate to have been around Jim Plunkett when we drafted him for the New England Patriots as a first pick. As a defensive coach in New York, I was there every day practicing against a guy like Joe Namath. Then in New Orleans we had Archie Manning, another great quarterback. If he had played for a team like the San Francisco 49ers, he probably would have accomplished what Joe Montana did. Then, of course, there was Brian Sipe with the Cleveland Browns.

But the guy I watched the most, the one who had the greatest impact on me, was Terry Bradshaw of the Pittsburgh Steelers. If you stood Terry Bradshaw and Brian Sipe side by side, they'd look like Bubba Smith, the great lineman, and Willie Shoemaker, the jockey. Terry had the physical attributes of a linebacker or a tight end. He was big and strong. He had an arm that could throw the football through the wind. When he threw a pass, it looked as if the ball had been shot out of a cannon. He had a jackhammer release.

He was an instinctive player. He could do what most quarterbacks couldn't and shouldn't do, and that's force the football into double coverage. Terry could do it. He had so much talent; he was the prototype. His talent often made up for mental mistakes he made on the field. Brian Sipe had to do everything right and do it by design. Bradshaw could recover from mistakes because of his strength and speed. He could throw into double coverage when there was no way Stallworth or Swann could be considered open. His arm strength and natural ability made the play. He was like Larry Bird, who seems to be able to hit the basket from any angle even if he's lying on the floor.

In 1979 in a game against the Steelers, we had about five minutes left in the fourth quarter, we had a 10-point lead, and I just knew that Bradshaw would jump out of a telephone booth like Clark Kent and do his version of Superman. Once during that game, we had Bradshaw trapped close to the Browns' side of the field. If we could sack him, they would have to punt, and we would get the ball. With our 10-point lead we should win the game, right? Terry came out of the pocket and looked up field, but he couldn't find an open receiver. He tucked the ball and ran like a runaway truck! I thought we would sack him.

Maybe a lot of people didn't know that Terry could run the ball about the way Franco Harris did. He didn't just go for first downs. On the few occasions when he did run the ball, you could tell he was going for six! As he ran by our bench, he was so close I could have reached out and touched him. In fact, it was all I could do to keep from tackling him because I knew he was going to make 20 or 25 yards. That's exactly what he did. He kept the drive going, scored a touchdown, tied the game, and finally beat Cleveland. It was Terry who beat us. He was all over the field, hitting critical passes on third down and running the ball to keep the drives alive. I stood on the sideline and watched Matt Bahr kick that field goal in the final minutes of overtime. Terry Bradshaw had gotten him into field-goal position. Terry whipped us. He made the big plays at the big time. The final score was 33–30.

Terry Bradshaw has to be one of the greatest quarterbacks who ever played the game, maybe the greatest. Why? Because he played in the modern-day Super Bowls, four to be exact. He won all four. Sure, they had great defense, great receivers, great runners, but without Bradshaw they never would have won so many championships. This is the biggest problem presently with the Steelers. No Bradshaw. He was the soul of the team. Out of that group of Steelers, I predict that eight or ten will be voted into the Hall of Fame. I also believe that at least six of them wouldn't make it if they hadn't played with Terry Bradshaw.

Terry was drafted as the number-one player, and the Steelers won the first game he quarterbacked. Then they lost the next sixteen straight games! Why? They didn't have the supporting cast. Terry was a young, inexperienced player from Louisiana Tech, a small school in Louisiana. A quarterback can't get the job done without good people around him.

But there's no way in the world you can win world championships without a great quarterback like Terry Bradshaw. To win championships, you need great players on both sides of the ball. But the quarterback remains the final link who puts it all together.

Jack Lambert was the quarterback of the Steeler defense. He was the hub in the wheel with ten spokes revolving around him and one of the very best ever to play linebacker. Jack was a second-round draft choice from Kent State who will join his teammate, Joe Greene, in the Hall of Fame. We had many confrontations with Jack because we played the Steelers twice each year. I got to know Jack pretty well when I coached him in the Pro Bowl in 1981.

When you sit down and talk with him man-to-man, he's very different from Jack Lambert the linebacker. He left pro football prematurely because of a very bad toe problem. He simply wouldn't continue to play unless he could play up to his own high standards. That made Jack different. Some players felt they could evaluate and apply their own degree of intensity as the situation dictated. Not Jack. He went all out, all the time. As a coach, I loved to see that in a player.

Every year, from 1978 on, Jack was a tremendous thorn in our side. Not only was he a great physical player, but he was very bright. Many a time I heard him from where I stood on the sideline, yelling and screaming at linebackers and defensive backs to make adjustments in their positions. Countless times he broke up our big passes and important runs. Lambert always seemed to be there to stop the play from being a big one. As a result we often had to kick a field goal instead of scoring 6 points that would have won the game. He was a very cerebral football player.

I remember our game in Pittsburgh in 1983 when Brian Sipe had dropped back to pass and he couldn't find an open receiver. He rolled out of the pocket and came toward our bench, but Jack Lambert caught him as he was going out of bounds and knocked him cold. Brian was finished for the day.

Ben Dreith, the referee, threw the flag and also threw Lambert out of the game. Ben Dreith is one of the best and most animated officials in the league. I was always happy to have Ben referee our Steeler games. His job as a referee is to protect the quarterback. Because of the Steelers' pass rush and intimidating style, Ben called many "roughing the quarterback" penalties. I kidded Ben when I met him on the field before the game. I told him, "Hey, Ben, if you're going to referee this game, I've got to call my wife and tell her to call the doctor. She'll need some tranquilizers if you're going to ref this game."

Lambert came right over to our bench and said to me, "Sam, that was not a cheap shot." After the game, Lambert came into our locker room to talk with Sipe. He really didn't intend to hurt Sipe. But when Lambert was involved in the heat and emotion of a game, that game to him was bigger than life, and he gave no quarter. Once the game was over, however, Jack was a very private person with a tremendous sensitivity.

We played another game against Pittsburgh in Cleveland in 1983 when Lambert did the same thing to Sipe and knocked him into our bench again. All our guys jumped him and hit him, and he finally ran out into the middle of the field. The referee threw him out of the game. He had caused Sipe to throw an interception, but the referee threw a flag and we kept possession of the ball. Whenever Lambert got thrown out of a game, it was a big help to us. When we were on the offense and Lambert was on the sideline, it was a comforting feeling. He had the respect of all the players.

Watching Lambert from the sideline as I did many times, I saw a physically tough and mentally alert player. Someone has said that deaf-mutes play the game of football with tremendous intensity and are great hitters. One of the reasons is that they can't hear the noise. Hearing the sounds of contact from the sideline is sometimes scary. You can also hear the sounds of people going after each other, screaming and groaning. Jack was an intense player who wasn't distracted by all that.

He was contagious. Young rookies who played with Jack played as much to please him as they did the coach. They knew they would hear from Jack if they didn't play up to the level that he felt was necessary to win. Even veteran players would feel his scorn at times. Jack played almost a decade with that great Steelers team.

I always felt that even if Jack Ham or Joe Greene or Donnie Shell or Mel Blount was out of the game, so long as Jack Lambert was there, the rest of the players would play to their optimum level. Coaches always talk about having a player who is like a coach on the field. That was Lambert. I always knew the Steelers would never beat themselves so long as Lambert was playing. Jack was both interesting and ominous to watch on the field because he was so animated. Every coach wants players like him. They don't come along every year.

When Lambert came out of college, many people didn't think he would make it because he appeared to be too long and tall but not heavy

WINNERS MAKE PLAYS ■ 199

enough. He was about six feet five and weighed about 210 pounds. His great innate strength gave him tremendous leverage, and he always seemed to be at the right place at the right time.

The moment a game started, Jack was like the conductor of the Cleveland Orchestra as he organized the line in front of him and the defense behind him. The defensive line and the linebackers always handled the running game while the defensive backs and the linebackers handled the passing game. For most of Jack's career he played in a four/three defense where he was the middle linebacker. He was the guy who orchestrated everything defensively and made the adjustments on each play. If we came out in an unusual formation or used a man in motion or anything exotic, Jack was the guy who had to get the word to the rest of the defense. And he almost always did.

The defense must respond as one. Communication is important. If there was a situation with third down and 6 yards to go and we threw the ball to Gregg Pruitt, Jack somehow got there to knock the ball down. If we had a back run out as a pass receiver, Jack seemed always to be able to run with him step for step and make the play. Or if we had a crucial third-down-and-one situation where we needed the first down to continue our drive, kill the clock, and get into field-goal position to win a game, Jack was always there on the line of scrimmage to stuff the play. He always made the big plays at important times. He shouldn't have been that good. He wasn't big enough. He was a throwback, the kind of player who should have played at Notre Dame in the 1940s. The guy simply loved to play football.

Jack didn't have much to say off the field. He was a private person. Sure, he had to negotiate his contract and got quoted in the newspaper once in a while. Seldom did he say anything negative. Once when he was asked what he thought about all the new rules to protect the quarterback, he replied, "From now on they oughta make sure the quarterbacks wear skirts!" But on the field he was as serious as they come. He didn't say things to please people; he said what he believed and felt strongly. Although I never had the pleasure of coaching Jack, I probably had more respect for him than most other players I ever watched. He's in a select category in my book.

The Steelers have lost a lot of great players in the last few years. Mel Blount, Jack Ham, Andy Russell, Dwight White, L. C. Greenwood, and Mean Joe Greene are gone. But what hurt them the most was losing Jack Lambert, future Hall of Famer. In all my years in professional football I never played against a guy, in any position, who was more of a dominating force than Jack Lambert, both physically and mentally. Jack was the complete player. If you could bottle what Jack Lambert had, it would be illegal! Yes, the Steelers were the best team of the 1970s. Four Super Bowl wins! They may go down in football history as the best team ever. Jack was selected on the second round. That's why the draft is a crapshoot. Sometimes it's better to be lucky than good.

Joe Greene was another fabulous player. He was a lot like Lambert, but he wasn't animated. He was a quiet, sleeping giant of a man. Joe helped Chuck Noll avert a possible racial issue on the team. When Joe Gilliam, the black quarterback, replaced Terry Bradshaw, he didn't work out so well, and Bradshaw was brought back as quarterback. There were rumblings about color and prejudice. Joe Greene was the person who provided the press with the truth: Joe Gilliam was given an opportunity with the Steelers, and he blew it.

I met Joe Gilliam when I was with the New Orleans Saints in Vero Beach, Florida, in 1977. Joe was out of Tennessee State where his father was the defensive coordinator. Joe was drafted initially by the Pittsburgh Steelers and was a very talented player. But he had a drug problem and was released by the Steelers.

That's when Coach Hank Stram gave him a second chance and signed him for the Saints when I was coaching for them. He showed up two days early for our training camp. He looked great and sounded very positive. He said he was finished with drugs. But when training camp actually started, Joe didn't show. We wondered where he was and investigated for a day or so. Coach Stram thought he had slipped again and wouldn't be able to handle the stress of training camp. But after a day or two, Joe called Hank Stram and said, "Coach, you won't believe this, but after I got settled in my room that first day I reported in, I was hitchhiking to downtown Vero Beach and got picked up by two girls. They accosted me and kept me in their room for three or four days."

Hank said, "I thought I'd heard 'em all. This gets the prize." When Hank hung up the phone and told us what Joe had said, we all rolled our eyes heavenward. So, Hank and all the rest of the coaches thought it would be best for the team to cut Joe, reasoning the way most coaches reasoned before drugs became so prevalent in the NFL. We agreed that our team was not a drug rehab center and that we simply couldn't handle any user on the club. We had to get people ready to play football. But to his credit, Hank Stram wanted to give Joe a chance. Joe had a tremendous talent and a great capacity to throw the football. We were concerned about Archie Manning, our quarterback, because he had been hurt. Archie was a great quarterback, but he just never had the chance to blossom because he never had a chance to play with great supporting players.

So we began practicing with Joe Gilliam in camp. It was my first opportunity to monitor a suspected drug user. I watched him closely every day, and it was soon obvious that Joe wasn't consistent. One day he would look great, and the next he wasn't crisp and alert. He didn't have the ability to read, recognize, and react. A quarterback has to be able to work his plan and make sure his plan is working. He has to hit the target between the two numbers on his receivers. He has to be on time. He has to see things and respond immediately. He has to know the offense inside out, call the plays, control the pulse of the other ten guys. He's the guy who directs the football team. He has to be the guy the other players look at in the huddle and say, "This guy can do it for me."

But Joe was like an EKG. He had highs and lows. He had brilliant moments, and then sometimes in a night practice he could hardly come out of the huddle. He could barely articulate in the huddle, and he just couldn't throw the football.

Then he began to wander around and miss meals and bed checks. He was found in other players' rooms. He was borrowing cars and money. He was doing the things I recalled later on when I was head coach of the Browns trying to understand the symptoms of a drug user. My experience with him was the beginning of drug awareness for me, but we didn't respond to it because we didn't know what to do. Hank had really tried to help Joe Gilliam. Hank even called Joe's father, but in the meantime Joe disappeared. Hank had to release him. Joe never made it back; he played in minor-league football after that and wasn't heard from again on the football field.

The tragedy was that Joe really had the talent to make it big in the NFL, but the demon drug pulled him aside. There was no drug program at that time. Maybe he could have weathered the storm if he could have been involved with an Inner Circle somewhere. There was no prevention, intervention, or aftercare for players in those days. Fortunately, Joe has recovered and is working for a drug rehab center in Nashville, Tennessee. I saw him not long ago at a drug symposium at the University of North Carolina where I spoke. Joe is helping other young people now and is healthy. Once again we have an example of someone who has been through the valley helping others who are mired down in their own valleys.

So it was Joe Greene who told the truth about Joe Gilliam when it was important for everyone to know the truth. Joe Greene was more of a leader in that episode than most people know. He was the father figure.

Joe Greene was a very real leader, but a very quiet one. He was just inducted into the Hall of Fame. He was the number-one draft pick one year after Terry Bradshaw was the first pick in his draft. In 1987 the Steelers hired Joe as a defensive line coach. I'm sure that most teams in the Central Division will be happy that he's just coaching instead of playing.

It was my good fortune to coach Franco Harris in 1981 in the Pro Bowl. When Franco was a senior at Penn State, he didn't have a great year in football. He wasn't even a heralded running back in the draft. The Steelers really didn't want to pick him. They were more interested in Robert Newhouse out of Houston University, who later went on to have a good career with the Dallas Cowboys. But someone in the Steelers organization knew Franco, and so they drafted him. Franco will go down in the record books as one of the greatest running backs in the history of the game. Again Lady Luck smiled on the Steelers. Another Hall of Fame pick.

Franco was an unusual back. He was big and strong, but if he was running the ball and saw that he was going to get hit and knocked out of bounds, he would step out. One of the signs of a great running back, like Walter Payton or Jim Brown, is his ability to elude tacklers. You could never really hit Franco. He wasn't always where he was "supposed" to be. He told me once that most of his great runs came when he cut back and left his blockers. Franco had a tremendous ability to evade tacklers. Even when he was trapped, he was able to come out of those traps and make yardage. Franco ran for 100 yards or more in all the big playoff games and Super Bowls. The Steel Curtain was important, Terry Bradshaw was important, but Franco was the one who could protect any lead the Steelers had because he could always pick up yardage to keep possession of the ball. He was also a very good receiver coming out of the backfield. He was a good athlete—period.

One year we had the Steelers stopped cold in Pittsburgh. Bradshaw threw twelve, count 'em, twelve passes to Franco. He ended up with over 100 yards gained by catching the football. In our preparations to play Pittsburgh, we always discussed Terry Bradshaw, of course, and Jack Lambert and the Steel Curtain, but we always acknowledged that we had to stop Franco Harris if we were going to win. If you let Franco run over you, it was all over that day. If you allowed a guy like Franco to gain over 100 yards, the quarterback could vary his offense and control the ball. Ball control comes from the running game, and that was Franco's department. Look at how long the Steelers enjoyed that because of Franco.

What was so remarkable about Franco was his character as a gentleman. He was very quiet and studious, very soft-spoken and involved in life outside of football. It's a shame that, at the end of his career, because of a contract squabble, he was not signed. Then he went to Seattle and was cut there.

At Pittsburgh, Franco was *the* guy of all the superstars. There was Franco's "army." The fans loved him. Once Franco and I talked at Cleveland, and he was very complimentary of me. He always seemed to say the right thing at the right time. Watching him crash through defenses and then sitting down to talk to that quiet man were an interesting contrast. He was a very good family man as well. He always talked about his mother and dad in the little New Jersey town where he was born. It's too bad he couldn't have ended his career at Pittsburgh. Franco's mother was Italian. His college coach was an old Brooklyn friend of mine, Joe Paterno. I was really proud of Franco's accomplishments and the way he handled them.

Football is a team sport. Players need one another. These outstanding winners needed something else as well. They needed and received outstanding coaching. As great as all these players were, they needed the coaches to bring out their highest potential. In the next chapter I'm going to talk about four men who are, in my opinion, the greatest coaches in the NFL today.

# CHAPTER THIRTY

# THE CHAIRMEN OF THE BOARD

**T**he four chairmen of the board in the NFL, listed alphabetically, are Tom Landry of the Dallas Cowboys, Chuck Noll of the Pittsburgh Steelers, Don Shula of the Miami Dolphins, and Bill Walsh of the San Francisco 49ers. They're my picks as the best because they've been involved in and won more Super Bowls than everybody else. But you have to ask if winning is the only measure of accomplishment. If it is, why don't Landry and Shula wear their Super Bowl rings? The reason they both give is that those Super Bowls happened in the past and the past is gone.

Bill Parcells won the Super Bowl in 1987 and is already hearing the "what have you done for me lately?" chorus. Nothing is deader than yesterday's newspaper. Once you've done it, you have to go out and do it all over again. The four chairmen of the board know this truth; they don't sit on their laurels.

The interesting thing about all four is that each of them had fantastic quarterbacks. Tom Landry had Roger Staubach, Chuch Noll had Terry Bradshaw, Don Shula had Johnny Unitas, Bob Griese, and Dan Marino, and Bill Walsh had Joe Montana. There was a cluster of stars on the Pittsburgh team, but Terry Bradshaw, in all the big games including playoff games and Super Bowl games, was *the* star. In the entire history of the NFL the teams who won the championships had great quarterbacks. They're the problem solvers and the guys who make the big plays. Bradshaw, Staubach, Montana, and Marino made the difference to their teams.

It's interesting to note what's happened since Pittsburgh lost Bradshaw and Dallas lost Staubach; neither team has made the playoffs regularly. They've even had losing seasons. Joe Montana's injury has hurt the San Francisco team. When Joe was healthy, they got to the summit twice and won both times. Don Shula is in a rebuilding year, but so long as you have a guy like Marino you have a chance.

Chuck Noll probably does more from the cerebral standpoint than most other coaches. He's very much the intellect. Prior to coming to Pittsburgh, he was an assistant coach on defense with Sid Gillman at San Diego and with Don Shula at Baltimore. When he arrived at Pittsburgh, he really developed the defense. Obviously they had a tremendous offense, but Chuck brought balance to the team. His experience included offense, defense, and special teams.

The great success at Dallas comes from stability. Tom Landry, Tex Schramm, the general manager, and Gil Brandt have been there a long time. Tom is the only coach Dallas has ever had. During the first seven years, Dallas never had a winning season. Then, Clint Murchison, the owner of the Cowboys, gave Landry a ten-year contract, even though Tom had a losing record. That gave them the continuity to build a team and an organization. That's why they've been to five Super Bowls and sixteen playoffs.

Don Shula has the Midas touch with one inch of velvet covering eleven inches of steel. He's had all those great quarterbacks. I believe Shula is the best coach in the NFL since Vince Lombardi. Bum Phillips said, "Don Shula can beatcha with his guys, and he can go to the other side of the field and beatcha with your guys!" That's the ultimate compliment from one coach about another.

Shula probably maximizes talent better than any coach. He gets people to play to the very best of their ability. All the great coaches have that knack. Lombardi had it, of course, and Shula does it better than anyone since Lombardi. Lombardi couldn't abide fumbling, but Shula hates it even more. That's a cardinal sin. He doesn't keep a fumbler around very long. All his players know that. Shula's expectation is that a player should *never* fumble. That's one way to get the best out of a player. It's the way he explains it to the players: "If you fumble, you're outta here!" He also has that all-important experience on both sides of the ball as well as the kicking game.

Bill Walsh is probably the most imaginative offensive football coach in the NFL. He's put together an offense engineered by Joe Montana that forces the defense to feel the pressure. He almost never allows the opposing defense to dictate to his offense. He's always on the offense. He's always coming up with creative ideas. Bill spent ten years with Cincinnati as an assistant to Paul Brown, but he left when Bill Johnson, another assistant, got the head coaching job. Bill went to San Diego as an assistant coach, then took a head coaching job at Stanford University. He told me then, "The reason I'm going to Stanford is that I want to do the best thing I can right now to enhance the possibility of my getting a head coaching job in the NFL." Bill had great success at Stanford and became head coach at San Francisco.

In 1981 Barb and I had dinner with Bill Walsh and his wife, Geri, at Palm Springs. He had just completed a second miserable year with San Francisco, and he was feeling mighty low. He moaned about how difficult it was at San Francisco. I really felt sorry for him. But all of a sudden his team took off, and they went to the Super Bowl in January of 1982 and beat Cincinnati. His first Super Bowl, and he won it against his old team. Then he took his team back a few years later and beat Miami.

The thing that makes the chairmen of the board great is that they've been to the summit; they've won the championship games. As Red Auerbach has said many times, "The only way to judge a team is if they win the world championships."

All four outstanding coaches know something so important that it seems simplistic: a quarterback has to have good protection, receivers must have a quarterback who can get the ball to them, and running backs must have linemen who can drive block and run block so that they can find the openings. Floyd Little, a three-time All-American at Syracuse, in his first year at Denver, couldn't gain 300 yards because he didn't have a good offensive line. O. J. Simpson suffered drastically at Buffalo until they got "The Electric Company," those five condominiums up on the line in front of "The Juice." They made O. J. an All-Pro, and he would be the first to say so.

All winning teams of the past have had great defensive lines. The defensive linemen don't have to worry about anybody else. All they have to do is disengage the guys in front of them and decide, of the four remaining backs, which guy has the ball and then go after him. A defensive lineman doesn't worry as much as the receiver, the offensive lineman, the running back, and the quarterback who are so dependent upon one another.

If you study the NFL from its inception, you'll find that the teams with great defensive lines—Pittsburgh and the Steel Curtain, for example—reached the summit. A defensive line, in the final four minutes, wins the game for you. To beat a great quarterback, you've got to have a great defensive line. A good rushing defensive line can do that.

Tom Landry had the Doomsday Defense. Don Shula had the No-Name Defense. The San Francisco linemen weren't named, but they were the most underrated part of the team. It was the defense that played so well in the final stretch of the season and in the Super Bowls. All these teams had great defensive lines and were able to pressure the opposing quarterbacks. History tells you that the NFL teams with the combination of a great quarterback and a great defensive line win the championships.

There are many ways to rate coaches. You can talk late into the night about it. But you can't win the Kentucky Derby with a jackass. A lot of coaches have the horses, but they can't ride them. You gotta have players. Shula has had players. A great football coach puts people in the best positions to help the team. He motivates them to maximize their talent and be as good as they possibly can be. Some players don't realize how much talent they have.

Shula motivates in many ways. He uses fear, incentive, and self-motivation. He's a product of all three. He's a martinet, a taskmaster, and can be tough and demanding. Anyone who has played for Shula will tell you that he's demanding from the very beginning of the season, yet he has a marked sensitivity. The players respect and, sometimes, fear Shula. The most important incentive in the NFL is to win the Super Bowl and wear the ring.

The winning players spend the entire off-season knowing they are the very best football team in the world. Once they get there, there is added incentive to stay. Shula has often said, "When you win it all, you cannot allow the players to forget the price they paid to get there." The Super Bowl winners go on a binge of banquets, speaking dates, endorsements, commercials, and contract negotiations. Then all of a sudden the off-season is over, and everybody has forgotten how they got there as champions. The lean and hungry ones become winners and then have to be careful not to get too fat and complacent. Fear and incentive are important motivators, but Shula probably uses self-motivation with his players better than anyone else.

For example, Nick Buoniconti was finished with the Boston Patriots when Miami got him for practically nothing. Shula traded for Paul Warfield, the number-one draft choice from Cleveland. He became a Hall of Famer. Jim Langer was a center who was waived by the Cleveland Browns and became a Hall of Famer with Miami under Shula. Bob Kuechenberg and Norm Evans, two unheralded offensive linemen, became part of that great offensive line that opened the holes for Larry Csonka, Mercury Morris, and Jim Kick and gave Bob Griese protection so he could get the ball up and away to Jim Mandich, Howard Twilley, and Paul Warfield.

Shula coached some great football players, but he also coached a lot of average players who became good under his coaching talents. He motivated many adequate players to become much better. Everybody around Shula became better players, whether it took fear, incentive, or self-motivation. He knew when to use each motivational tool.

Shula demanded and got the very best out of his players every year at all levels. Even during his lean, transitional years between Griese's retirement and Marino's drafting, he got the most from his men. Five quarterbacks were picked ahead of Marino that year. Yet Marino was an instant success and went to the Super Bowl. Shula saw to it that he got the best pass protection in the NFL. He demanded it, and he got it. Marino became a star even though he was picked after five other quarterbacks were picked. The difference in his development was Shula. That's what coaching is all about.

Shula is well organized, uses good judgment, has made judicious trades, has drafted well without making many mistakes, and has developed his choices to the fullest. He gets people to play from the soles of their feet to the tops of their heads, from locker room to locker room.

Everybody knows that Miami rarely makes mistakes. Shula has drafted guys who rarely make mistakes. It is often said of Shula, "His teams won't beat themselves. If you beat them, then you deserve the win." His players give the best they've got all the time. As long as Shula is at Miami, they'll always be a threat. They'll get to the Super Bowl again. That's what Shula is all about. That's what the four chairmen of the board are all about. They win the big ones, the championships. But any of them will tell you that you've got to have players. To get good players, you've got to draft smart and, sometimes, draft lucky.

# CHAPTER THIRTY-ONE

# THE DRAFT

**T**he college football draft is virtually a crapshoot. It's like going to Las Vegas and rolling the dice. All the measurable attributes—height, weight, speed, arm length, and the span of a man's hand—are important. Long arms give leverage to an offensive lineman. The span of a defensive lineman's hand is important so that he can grab the offensive player by the jersey, jerk him, and push him aside. If a defensive lineman can cause the offensive lineman to move his head, his body will be turned. It's like checking the teeth of a horse. These things can be measured.

The problem is that there are no absolutes, and sometimes the exceptions are fantastic. You just never know what you might get when you draft a player because you can't measure motivation, intensity, and competitive drive. You find out about those things after the fact, after you buy the horse. The great ones have something called "heart." It's like an exercise EKG. You don't really know what you've got until you see them under stress. Red Auerbach said it best when he was asked how in the world he was able to win seventeen championships. He answered, "Good people." You can manage things, but you must lead people.

The draft is an interesting thing for a coach. You go out and visit schools, colleges, and universities all over the United States. Information, as I've often said, is like eggs—the fresher the better. You watch films until you're bleary-eyed. You grade the players as you watch every move they make on film. You watch them practice; you watch them play their scheduled games; you talk to their trainers, coaches, family, teachers, and counselors. You give them intelligence tests. You measure every single measurable thing you can think of. In the final analysis, it's a matter of using experience and judgment when an organization drafts a player.

Where does the experience come from? Experience! For example, Gil Brandt of the Dallas Cowboys has been with that organization for twenty years as director of player personnel. Al Davis of the Los Angeles Raiders has been there as a coach who walked the sideline, a general manager, and now an owner. Experience! The first coach Davis hired was John Rauch who took the team to the Super Bowl. The second coach he hired was John Madden who took them to the Super Bowl. The third coach he hired was Tom Flores who took them to the Super Bowl twice. Here's a team that has never fired a coach. Red Auerbach's coaches, with one exception, have won world championships. Red Auerbach and Al Davis are kingmakers. The Los Angeles Dodgers have a farm system and an organization that produce consistent winners. Don Shula has been with the Miami Dolphins for twenty years. Experience! Chuck Noll of the Steelers has been there almost twenty years. Tom Landry of the Dallas Cowboys has been there ever since the team was first organized. Experience! Organization! Judgment! Like insurance actuaries, they just don't make as many mistakes as the other teams make.

Every time another team hires a new coach there are a lot of personnel and coaching changes because new brooms do sweep clean. But it takes an old broom to get in the corners. I decided that, yes, I would listen to everybody, but we needed to see the draft prospects ourselves. Would you believe that, in 1978, people came to me and said Brian Sipe couldn't win for us? We said we would find out for ourselves. Ozzie Newsome was a split end in the wishbone formation in college. We said let's find out for ourselves if he can be a tight end. Reggie Rucker was "washed up," they said. Dave Logan was going to be a tight end and had never played. Tom DeLeone, a center who was cut by eight or ten teams, eventually went to the Pro Bowl as a result of his play with the Browns. We went to see these guys for ourselves.

I've been to eighteen drafts for five different teams. To work the draft right, you have to study the prospects for an entire year. You start with as many as seven thousand names, work it down to about seven hundred, and then boil that down to about three hundred. Those are the ones you concentrate on. Today, with the drug and alcohol problems, you have to dig even deeper into the past of players.

The first and second rounds are the most exciting. After that you might as well go to the Manhattan directory and throw darts at the names. The first- and second-round choices are the ones who will probably stay with you the longest. Drafting players is like investing in equipment. You have to keep it working long enough to get your investment back and then enjoy some profits. The profits are closely tied with championships. Right now Ozzie Newsome, Hanford Dixon, Clay Matthews, and Bernie Kozar are examples of superstars who are going to win for you.

On draft day you have all your prospects rated by position. Then you huddle with your coaches and rerate the players, not by position, but by order of importance. Someone will say there's a receiver at Stanford; someone else will mention a guy at Michigan and another one at Florida. Then we consider who is the best receiver of the bunch. Next we ask ourselves if we have a better chance of getting to the championships with a linebacker like Jack Lambert or a defensive end like Mark Gastineau or a running back like Earl Campbell or an offensive lineman like John Hannah. We ask ourselves who is the best player, regardless of position, on any given NFL team. We think about all the existing teams and their outstanding players to use as models for our draft choices. We try to find a pattern, but it's impossible. If you would list the best player in all the NFL teams in the United States, it would defy explanation.

Beauty, truly, is in the eye of the beholder. Everybody views the draft prospects differently. As the names come off the board, you see names being picked that you thought might not be picked at all. Other surprises include those names everybody talked about before the draft, but they stay up there a long time. Then you wonder what other people know that you don't know. Or if you pick up a guy at a bargain rate late in the draft, somebody will say you stole him. It's like handicapping horses. Everybody's got reasons for picking names.

There's always the time crunch on draft day, too. As each name disappears from the board—sometimes as a surprise to everybody—you have to quickly reorganize and reshuffle. You don't have all day. It's like a dealers' automobile auction. They run them through fast, and you have to make a decision. Judgment, organization, and experience are absolutely necessary to draft players successfully.

I remember one director of player personnel who always went to the bathroom when the final selection was being made. Being in that board room is like being in a war room. It's like being in there with the president and all the military leaders and everybody wants to know who's going to push the button when the red telephone rings. Somebody has to make a decision about which players to draft. What it comes down to is a consensus. Everybody has to agree that the draftees fill the bill where the team has the greatest need. You have to be very careful about getting the names right, too.

In 1979 the Browns had two second-round draft choices. With the first draft choice we selected Sam Claphan, an offensive tackle from the University of Oklahoma. On the second pick we chose Lawrence Johnson, a cornerback from Wisconsin. As soon as you make the selections, the director of player personnel or the secretary contacts the player, who is usually waiting at home for the telephone call. Then Art Modell talks to him and welcomes him to the team. The director tells him about coming into a minicamp and gives him all the details, making sure the player isn't going to sign with a Canadian team. Then the head coach is the final person to talk to the new draftee. As in Lawrence's case, for example, I got on the phone and said, "Lawrence, congratulations."

He said, "Coach, I can't tell you how excited I am about being drafted by the Cleveland Browns."

"We're happy about you, Larry. You've got an excellent chance to play for us. We need you in that position."

"Hey, Coach, I'm really excited. I didn't expect to be drafted until about the tenth round! I thought I might even be a free agent."

I thought to myself, *How can Larry be thinking this way?* We had rated him as one of the top cornerbacks in the United States. He was a sprinter at the University of Wisconsin, and he's telling me that he's surprised at how high we picked him. A chilling thought hit me and slid through my body. Had we made some horrible mistake? Why would Larry be so elated?

When I put the phone down, I looked at Art Modell and said, "I never heard a draftee so excited as Larry. He almost came through the phone. It doesn't add up, Art."

Art said, "Why shouldn't he be delighted to sign with the Browns?"

"Yeah, but this guy, I don't know, Art. We'd better double-check. Maybe we made a mistake in our research. Maybe we got the wrong guy."

I asked Tommy Prothro to check the name, and sure enough, there were two Larry Johnsons. I yelled to everybody, "Mamma Mia, we just called and congratulated the wrong guy! We drafted the wrong

Larry Johnson! Quick, you guys, make some phone calls! Get this straightened out before the press hear about it!''

As it turned out, there was another Larry Johnson who was a defensive lineman for the University of Mississippi. That was the guy we had on the telephone, not the Larry Johnson we thought we drafted. The lid blew off! We had drafted the wrong player! But after a few frantic phone calls, we learned that we had, indeed, drafted the right Lawrence Johnson but had telephoned the wrong Larry Johnson. Finally we contacted the right Lawrence Johnson, and everybody breathed a sign of relief. Tommy Prothro might have gotten fired that day if we had drafted the wrong player. So, draft day is exciting, but you'd better be prepared when the bidding starts!

Sometimes, no matter how well prepared you think you are, things can change at the last minute and throw you into a panic. That's what happened to me on March 26, 1987.

# CHAPTER THIRTY-TWO

# THE GREAT DEBATE

After I was fired in 1984, NBC, CBS, and ABC called me to audition for a broadcasting position. I signed with NBC because I had worked for them in the past as a part-time consultant.

On Thursday, March 26, 1987, I flew to New York City to tape a half-hour special for an NBC show at the invitation of Bob Trumpy, the moderator, and Larry Fleisher, the attorney for the professional basketball players' associations. I had been asked to debate this gentleman on the question of mandatory drug testing for professional athletes. I was to make the case for testing while Larry Fleisher was to oppose it. His position was based on the Fourth Amendment to the Constitution, which guarantees freedom from invasion of privacy. This debate is now raging from the Pentagon to college campuses.

In the news was the story of Simone LaVant, a young diver from Stanford University who had refused to be tested for drugs. She was the only one of fifteen thousand athletes in the NCAA who would not submit to a drug screen. Her case was upheld by the California Supreme Court. She appeared on an hour-long "Phil Donahue Show" during the week of March 22, 1987, with John Toner, athletic director of the University of Connecticut and also president of the NCAA, and with an ACLU attorney who represented her.

Of course, I was intensely interested in this question because the mandatory drug screen had contributed to the success of the Inner Circle. Drug testing is just part of the cure, but it does convey to everyone that there is a problem. Each of the players involved in the Inner Circle desperately needed those two drug screens each week. They had to remain clean, and they knew it. But we knew also that they weren't going to make it in the early phases of the program without tough love. A clean drug test was the only guarantee that they were telling the truth and were on their way to credible sobriety one day at a time.

I thought back to the early days of the Inner Circle in the fall of 1982 when we discovered that one Inner Circle participant would stay clean each week and urinate in the bottles for all the other players. Sometimes they would bring clean urine in and then switch bottles.

When I found out what they were doing, I was livid. I wanted to kick them all into Lake Erie. How dumb did they think we were? Like my dad said, "I was born at night, but not last night." I wanted to choke them individually. I tasted the despair that parents of autistic children must feel when those children constantly beat themselves. I just couldn't believe they would come to meetings week after week, smile at me, and tell me how great everything was going since they got "clean." These guys looked at us and lied right through their teeth.

I was disgusted with the entire program. I wanted to chuck it all. Who needed this? I might as well flog myself. Everyone was down except the doctor. His experience brought us through the crisis. I thought about all that as I prepared to appear on national television to discuss mandatory drug screens for professional athletes.

The NBC appearance fit in with my schedule, which included a speaking date in New York City at the Downtown Athletic Club. I felt good about the debate because I knew a lot about the subject and cared a great deal about it, also. I had been on ESPN with Roy Firestone in Los Angeles, and I had a chance to sing the praises of the Inner Circle. Now I was going to have a chance to do more.

When I arrived at Runyon's Restaurant, where sports shows are often taped, I learned that attorney Larry Fleisher couldn't keep the date but that an ACLU attorney would fill in. The subject was a hot one. The day before I got there, George Young, the general manager of the New York Giants, and Lee Steinberg, an agent from the Los Angeles area who represented professional athletes, had debated it. The NBC people apparently wanted to keep digging into the subject because there were such strong feelings on both sides.

I arrived at 4:30 in the afternoon and was met by a man named Stu Black. He said, "Sam, I'm sorry we couldn't get the ACLU attorney."

"No problem, Stu."

"We thought we had someone else from the ACLU, but that fell through, also. But we did get you an opponent."

"Hey, whoever you got is all right with me. What's this gentleman's name?"

"F. Lee Bailey."

"For a minute there I thought you said F. Lee Bailey!"

"I did."

"*The* F. Lee Bailey?"

"Yep."

"Tell me you're joking, Stu."

"It's for real, Sam. He's here already."

"Good heavens, I'll be creamed!" For a few seconds I considered diving out a window to escape. F. Lee Bailey! Horrors! In about twenty minutes I was scheduled to go in front of the cameras and face the Clarence Darrow of the 1980s. There was no time to think. I couldn't even find a place to hide. Had I known who I was to face I might not have shown up. But it was too late to duck out now. It would be like me as a high-school coach debating Vince Lombardi on how to run the sweep back in the 1960s. I was completely overwhelmed. David and Goliath came to mind—only this time I didn't have a script. Nobody knew how my mind was working during that period of about three minutes. It was panicsville.

Just then Lee walked in. There he stood, right in front of me. I was awed. He was a living legend, a Hall of Famer in the legal profession. But he put me at ease immediately. I blurted out something about his famous Sam Shephard murder case, and he was very gracious. Bob Trumpy and I were like two little kids talking to this famous man just prior to the show.

Finally we went upstairs and hooked up all the mikes in readiness for the cameras. We had about six minutes until air time. As each minute passed, I got more nervous. I was about to go on national television opposite F. Lee Bailey himself. What had I gotten into? At about three minutes to air time I said to myself, *Self, cool it. You know a lot about this subject. Don't worry. Bailey will talk about the law and the Constitution. He hasn't dealt with the nitty-gritty of the drug issue. He's a big-picture man.* Then I prayed, "Lord, I've got a golden opportunity to make a fool out of myself in about two minutes. But I've also got a chance to relay a very important message, not only to coaches and players on every level from Pop Warner to the NFL but also to parents all over America. Lord, You know we're at war in this country and that 90 percent of the world's cocaine is consumed here. Use me, Lord, for Your glory."

When the lights went on, all my anxieties disappeared. Lee Bailey was a gentleman, and I believe both of us made good presentations. It was scheduled to be aired nationally on the weekend of April 11, 1987. Lee stressed the constitutional side of the question and maintained that professional athletes were not role models. Of course, I felt strongly that young boys really look up to the pro athletes and want to be just like they are, both on and off the field. I suggested that we could go to the nearest school yard and find young boys who wanted to model themselves after Julius Erving, Reggie Jackson, Ozzie Newsome, or Michael Jordan. Professional athletes are special persons.

Sure, I expressed my concern about constitutional rights and invasion of privacy. But I was more concerned about Len Bias's parents and Don Rogers's mother and about young people all over America who were committing suicide. I told him that we didn't need to stand behind some law in the country as much as we needed to stop the bleeding. Mandatory drug testing may not cure the problem, but it might help recreational users to stop. It will uncover them in time to help them. It will also uncover the addicts who might otherwise be too far down the drainpipe to stop themselves. Most important of all, it might prevent young players from starting the use of drugs.

Lee made the first statement, and I came back with a pretty strong statement. Then there was a commercial break. Lee looked at me and smiled. "You're gonna pay for that." I'm very glad he smiled. For the next half hour we went at it.

Of course, Lee Bailey is as much against drugs as any thoughtful person, but he still feels strongly about our rights in America. I was grateful for the appearance with a man of his stature. I left the scene feeling that it would cause many people to think the issue through and that it would be good for our young people to hear and to ponder.

In my view, all the talk in the world and all the effort put forth—including prevention, intervention and aftercare—aren't enough. Those are necessary steps, but they take you only so far. There has to be another ingredient without which there will be no lasting cure. In medicine we have the help of dedicated professionals. But still more is needed. I've learned in my own life that Christ's words are as true today as they ever were: "without Me, you can do nothing." Until I learned that, nothing ever happened in my life that had lasting fulfillment. This truth was affirmed to me once again in a most unlikely place. I discovered it afresh in attempting to minister to some of society's "throw away" kids who are located just fifteen minutes' drive from Cleveland Municipal Stadium.

# CHAPTER THIRTY-THREE

# TWO LIVES:
# ONE WE LIVE,
# ONE WE LEARN

Joe Abraham, the staff minister for Youth for Christ in the inner city of Cleveland, had often talked to me while I was the Browns' coach. He ministered to my needs when I got fired. I was tempted to hide in a closet because of my bitterness and shame. Everything I had worked all my life for had been taken away. I had climbed the corporate ladder for twenty-nine years, and suddenly, someone had said I was no longer competent enough to handle the football team. I thought back to Harry Truman's words: "The way in which you endure that which you have to endure is really more important than the crisis itself." I had been thinking about that a great deal when Joe Abraham called and wanted to have breakfast with me.

At the restaurant, Joe said, "Sam, you can go out and speak at a lot of places. You can speak for twenty minutes or half an hour, but that's not enough. Why don't you consider coming into the inner city of Cleveland to teach at a junior high school or a high school?"

"I don't know, Joe. I'm not sure what I want to do right now. Maybe I could do something like that for a while. I just don't know." I thought of the truism that a good friend will sometimes tell you things you don't especially want to hear.

Joe continued, "Sam, you just can't go out now and speak forty or fifty times a year. Last year I asked you to speak about the drug issue at a Glenville High School student assembly at the end of the year. And you did."

"Yeah, and it wasn't easy. They've heard everything that needs to be heard about drugs. Frankly, they know more than I do or any drug expert who ever spoke to them."

"I know."

"But, Joe, at least I really cared about those kids. But for the grace of

God, there go I. I don't know how else I escaped it growing up where I did."

"Sam, when you spoke to those kids, they listened. You had an impact on them, but it was for just that one day. Twelve hours later they wouldn't see you again. If you really want to get involved in any kind of ministry, you need to go back and follow up. That's what I've had to do for eleven years. There was just a little fruit at first. I had to keep going. If you go out and make a speech, you're the apple. If you keep going back, you're the seed that produces the apples."

"That's interesting, Joe. I need to think it through." Actually I was a little annoyed at Joe for saying such things to me. After all, I was doing a lot for God, making all those speeches, telling how God had changed my life. But Joe was suggesting that it wasn't enough. Nobody likes to be weighed and found wanting, and I was no exception. After I thought about it awhile, I saw that I could, in my own way, do what the recovered drug addict can do. I could show that I had walked through my own kind of dark valley and I could still be grateful to God. The attitude of gratitude. Maybe God was giving me a chance to give it away, to share with others.

I thought back to how I started out as a teacher in New York City making four thousand dollars a year. Now I had economic freedom, and I had a chance to go into the inner city one day a week and teach. I took stock. In 1956 I was not a believer. Now, some thirty years later, I was. Now I was better equipped as a teacher. It began to make some sense to me.

I looked in the book of Psalms and asked the Lord to point out the right way for me to go. Joe and I prayed about it together, and then we went to Glenville High School. I felt like asking God, "Are You sure? The inner city? Couldn't You start me out with a nice suburban school, Lord?"

Our first meeting was with Mr. Pfeifer, the principal. I cleared my throat and said, "Mr. Pfeifer, we'd like to help your kids if we could."

"Let me get this straight. You two gentlemen want to come in here to Glenville High School and teach?"

Both Joe and I smiled and said, "That's right."

"Why would you want to do this?"

Joe said, "We want to help them. They'll come if Sam shows up. They'll come out of curiosity if nothing more."

Pfeifer smiled, "That's for sure. But what is it you want to teach them?"

I said, "We don't know what we want to do exactly because we don't know your curriculum. We thought you might tell us what the needs are and how we might fit in.

"I'd like to give it a shot. Who knows, maybe I'll get fired from Glenville, too!"

"Well, it's an intriguing proposition. We have some youngsters here who do not regularly come to school. We have some very tough kids here. Some of them are difficult to motivate. They've given up. They have very little hope. Let me give it some thought. Let me call you in a few days after I've had an opportunity to think it over.

"Gentlemen, if you can get some of our youngsters motivated, that's all right with me."

*Motivation* was the key word, as it turned out. When Mr. Pfeifer called us later, that's the subject we were assigned—Motivation and Life. Neither Joe nor I kidded ourselves about why they had let us come to Glenville. What got them to agree was not because it was Sam Rutigliano or Joe Abraham or Youth for Christ or any kind of ministry; it was simply because they could get the former head coach of the Cleveland Browns to come one day a week, and that would draw the interest of the kids. That would get them to school. I didn't care what the motivation was. The only important thing was to begin following up the way Joe suggested. The greatest thing was to be able to give it away. To whom much has been given, much is expected.

Mr. Pfeifer said, "We'll put a group of difficult students together for you. They don't care a great deal about school. We are having difficulty motivating them. Each one of them has some big problem in his or her life. Some of them walk onto the school grounds in the mornings and haven't had anything to eat since noon the previous day. Some of the young girls are pregnant."

Next we visited Mr. Freillino, the principal of the junior high school. All he wanted to talk about was football, and all we wanted to talk about was our ministry. He decided to do the same thing as Mr. Pfeifer. He, too, put together a group of unmotivated kids. What could the administrators lose? So there I was, thirty years after being a teacher at George Westinghouse Vocational High School in Brooklyn, in a very similar situation.

One day I was teaching our new class at Glenville about partnerships. I asked the class, "Suppose you were going to attempt to walk across Niagara Falls on a tightrope. Anybody knows that you don't attempt something like that unless you've practiced it a lot, right? One mistake and it's all over; you're dead. Suppose I asked you if you really believed that I could make it across. Then, suppose I asked you if you trusted me enough to ride across on my back."

One of the students said, "You're outta your mind, you're crazy!"

I said, "I agree with you. If you asked me that same question, I'd give you the same answer."

Then suddenly, in the back of the room, two young guys squared off. Pancho (not his real name), a young man with a fire raging inside himself, was fighting with another young man. They were screaming and cursing at each other. All the bad language came out. I heard Pancho use *that* word on the other kid. I tried to step in, and Pancho's eyes blazed at me with contempt as he stabbed his finger in the air and said the same thing to me.

For a few seconds, I was no longer standing in that room. I was back at George Westinghouse Vocational High School facing the young man once again who had defied my authority thirty years ago. The scene played itself out in my mind as I felt my adrenaline preparing me for action. I saw myself as a young man, standing in the aisle of the classroom, itching to slug the young man and finally doing it. I saw him fall in a limp heap at my feet. I felt the surge of satisfaction pour through my veins. I found myself wanting to do the same thing to Pancho. And then I remembered the principal's words, echoing through the time and space of thirty years, "That's what he deserves, but it's not what he needs."

Now, here I was again, in another galaxy, in another city, in another classroom, in the same situation. A face-off, one-on-one, between rebellion and authority, the cause and effect of almost all human misery and suffering. I felt that gentle balm inside my chest, the peace that passes all understanding, keeping me calm. Even more, I felt a deep sorrow and sympathy for Pancho. But at the same time, I felt all the feelings a challenged man feels when threatened. Both influences pulled at me in those few short seconds while I gathered myself together. Every eye in the room was on me. The air was crackling with electricity as everyone waited for my reaction. Time stopped and hung there like a camera still-shot. Nobody moved. Sam Rutigliano, former NFL coach, was being called out by a raging young man who didn't care what happened next; a young man nobody cared about; a young man who had nothing to lose by tweaking the beak of a sports celebrity in front of his peers.

I smiled at Pancho and said, "Hey, you speak the language very well. I want you to know that thirty years ago a student said that to me in my first week as a new teacher in Brooklyn, New York, and I knocked him cold. I can't kid you, Pancho, because that's what I feel like doing to you right now, but I'm not gonna do it. I want you to know that, regardless of what you think or how you feel, I'm here right now because I love you."

The two combatants stopped dead in their tracks and spun around toward me. Their eyes told me their thoughts, their disbelief, their cynicism. They had turned around to verify their certainty that I was being sarcastic. They searched my eyes like two young tigers fighting, who pause and stare only long enough to read the mood of their approaching keeper.

Quietly I said, "You heard me. I love you, and I think you're worthwhile. You and everybody else in this room are important. Joe Abraham and I care about you. That's why I told you the story about Niagara Falls because my next thought for you is that Jesus Christ would walk across with you. You could go on His back, and He would go across. He would go across on your back when nobody else in the world would. You and I have nobody else—mother, father, brother, or sister—who would make that kind of commitment to us!"

At a time like that, you simply can't whip out your Bible and start quoting Scripture. If you did, they would call downstairs and say, "Hey, get an ambulance quick and bring two guys with white jackets because we got a guy up here who's nuts!" Sometimes Bible lessons are better shown than read.

We told the principals that we were going to be spiritually based and that's the way we applied our lessons. The reason they allowed us to do it was because they had tried everything and had given up. Even the ACLU let us alone. If they had been so inclined, they would have been in there to throw us out before we put our first objective on the blackboard. The moment somebody finds out what we're doing, we're gonna get thrown out.

But the important thing about it at this writing is that we're still there. Now if either Joe or I can't make the scene one day, the kids inquire about us. They say, "Where's Joe? Where's Sam?" We can't accomplish miracles in forty minutes once a week, but at least we've seen changes, changes that will have lifelong effects. I've seen kids go for knives, guns, whatever they think they can bring from home to get even with some other kid. I've seen total, uncontrolled rage erupt right in the classroom. But after a few months, the kids didn't get up and storm out of the classroom if they got mad at some other kid. They hung in there. Sure, they yelled at each other and used all the words, but they stayed in their seats and didn't try to murder each other. Hey, that's progress! Love, even tough love, worked with my two kids that day.

I think with great wonder that I'm only fifteen minutes away from Cleveland Municipal Stadium where I used to have a captive audience. About 80,000 people watched me from the stands. On "Monday Night Football," maybe 80 million watched me on television. Now I'm in front of 35 incorrigible kids who might as well have terminal cancer, who have been on the road to nowhere, to Hopeless Gulch. I've asked myself, *What hath God wrought?* After six months, I've realized that some of these castoffs look forward to our class one day each week. Why? Because nobody else cares about them.

So maybe only one or two make it. It's worth it. How much is one life worth? It depends on which end of the gun you're looking down! There's no Super Bowl ring, there's no big contract, no endorsements, no prestige, and no interest from the media. It's great! We could have given up on these kids, but by the grace of God, we didn't, just as we didn't give up on the members of the Inner Circle. Would I do it all over again? You bet I would.

As for the future, I can't say. For now I'm very busy with speaking engagements all over the United States and in some foreign countries, television contracts with NBC and ESPN, book contracts, and many opportunities for ministry. More important, I have time for my family now for the first time in almost thirty years. How much more fulfilled can a man be?

Every Wednesday, Joe Abraham and I sit in his car and pray before going to be with the kids at school. But greatest of all, we know the Lord is with us and He cares. I can't wait to see what He has for us to do next. Barb and I trust Him for all of life. As a head coach in the National Football League, I always tried my very best to please the owner. While that's certainly important, I now see that all my efforts should be directed toward pleasing the Owner of the entire universe. I'll take my chances with Him. He continues to love me—even when I lose games. He took the pressure off when He promised never to fire me!

### *"an inside look at a man who . . . knows how to win"*

Sam Rutigliano knows something about pressure. But more importantly, he knows how to deal with pressure. I have heard Sam speak, and he tells it like it is. He does so in this book as well, and I would recommend it to everyone, as we all face pressures every day of our lives.

*Pressure* gives an inside look at a man who not only knows how to win on the field, but knows how to win in life.

> Jerry Falwell
> *Thomas Road Baptist Church*

### *"he truly cares for his players"*

Sam Rutigliano goes above and beyond the ordinary responsibility of being a coach. He truly cares for his players and takes steps to help educate them not only in football, but also in the many problems encountered in life.

> Don Shula
> *Head Coach and Vice President, Miami Dolphins*

### *"autobiography at its best"*

Sam Rutigliano is a passionate man. *Pressure* epitomizes his passion for winning, for integrity, for caring, for excellence, and for spirituality. This is autobiography at its best. Sam and I grew up together, and we both became football coaches. Believe me when I tell you this is an insider's book about football and the accompanying pressures on coaches, players, owners, and their families.

> Joe Paterno
> *Head Football Coach, Pennsylvania State University*

### *"riveting and powerful description of pressure"*

No question about it, Sam Rutigliano understands pressure. He gives a riveting and powerful description of pressure in the NFL. More thrilling to me, however, is the way Sam communicates that God can take the pain out of pressure. If you are concerned about pressure in your life, don't miss Sam's book.

> Joe Gibbs
> *Head Coach, Washington Redskins*